THE ART

OF STONE HEALING

WHERE THE PAST MEETS THE PRESENT

A dynamic therapy that can lead
to well-being and spiritual growth.

~ Sonia Alexandra ~

First paperback edition 2004. Printed in U.S.A.

Cover design by Gail Pocock

Text set in Bookman Old Style.

Manufactured in the United States of America.

ISBN 0-9758711-0-2 First edition

Library of Congress Control Number 2004095034

This book is available at special quantity discounts to use as in training programs. Please write to:

Sonia Alexandra
4521 North Dixie Highway
Boca Raton, Florida 33431

Celestial

O

O

(Cosmic Energy)

O

O

The Stone's

The Pathway

O

O

O

(Earth Energy)

Terrestrial

Begin With Nature's Gift

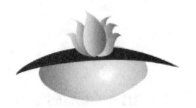

In India, the Lotus Blossom is the
most important symbol of spirituality.

* * *

The most exquisite of all callings, the search for the self, permeates every level of society. The health of the mind, body and spirit is an expression of the balanced life we all seek.

Our greatest challenge is to pursue our true self.

Stone healing aids us in this process, helping us to discover the sacred place within the internal core of our being: the "I am" within.

We discover our true authentic self, our source, this unbounded energy reconnecting with the life source.

The Art of Stone Healing

To Alexander,

my greatest blessing.

Embrace your journey, my son.

* * *

The Art of Stone Healing

Dear God,

Allow us to see the world
with the symbolic sight
of spiritual awareness.

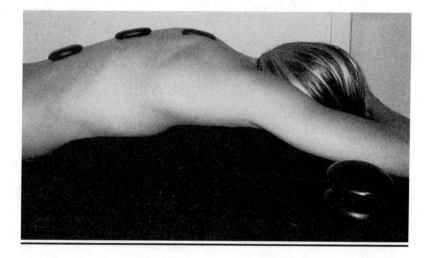

Where the past meets the present.

* * *

<u>The Water Course Way</u>

As the soft yield of water

cleaves obstinate stone,

So to yield with life

solves the insoluble.

To yield, I have learned,

is to come back again.

But this unguarded lesson,

this easy example,

is lost on Man.

Lao Tsu

The Art of Stone Healing

CONTENTS

To almost every group of people some sort of stone played a central role in their beliefs either medicinal, spiritual or as a symbol of power.

* * *

To ancient people, crystals were sacred gifts. As time went on, they retained their magical and spiritual qualities. Priests, medicine men, rulers and shaman wore these powerful gems as symbols of spiritual and temporal authority.

* * *

ACKNOWLEDGEMENTS

Foremost to my son Alex, who recently lost Josephine, his wife and the love of his life, after a lengthy illness: Thank you for teaching me the true meaning of unconditional love.

I also wish to acknowledge those whom I admire and who have greatly influenced my life, beginning with . . .

Robert, who gifted me thirty years ago with Napoleon Hill's book, *Think and Grow Rich.* Its cover reads, "This book could be worth a million dollars to you." Well, it certainly was worth that to me, and more. The applied principles within that little book changed the course of my life. Here is an example of how transformative and change-inducing a simple book can be in influencing our lives in a majority of ways.

Louise Hay, eighteen years ago I brought your book home after attending a Unity Church service. *You Can Heal Your Life* was a catalyst to a higher level of personal growth. Thank you, Miss Hay, you were truly inspiring.

Then along came Anthony Robbins when I was ready and receptive. His message was loud and clear: Positive Thinking.

Spiritual Deepak Chopra and his insights: Thank you for making a tremendous difference in my life.

And awesome Oprah, what can I say? You are influencing the world, my lady.

Mr. Donald Trump: What a phenomenal comeback.

Both Sting and Bono: Such tremendous humanitarian efforts. I admire and thank you.

And finally, my great appreciation to Marcel Patenaude, my business partner, who challenged me to be a stronger businessperson and to no longer let my emotions rule.

INTRODUCTION

This book is devoted to all traditions whose humanitarian efforts and dedication bring balance and compassion into our world and with it transformation on a multitude of levels.

"This is where the Past meets the Present."

We will examine the ancient remedy of Stone Therapy, addressing the profound spiritual disconnection among our physical body, heart and soul. We will see how we can use Stone Therapy to reconnect and integrate these disparate entities both internally and externally. I will show the reader how to reconnect, through deep relaxation and balance, directly to our innermost self, into our highest level of being, into the silence within.

There are obvious and subtle factors ever-present that are responsible for disconnecting us from our bodies. The ever-accelerating pace of our lives causes profound alienation from our selves, others and nature. With so many distractions, many of us have little time for personal relationships, prayer or meditation. But this is the rich soil in which we can truly grow spiritually.

The beginning practices of Stone Therapy focus primarily on the physical and energetic aspects of the human body and mind. We will explore deep inner emotional and spiritual blockages, how the body and mind are influenced and affected by multi-dimensional energy systems and how these changes affect us in relation to Stone Therapy.

These beginning practices lay the foundation for the Intermediate and Advanced Stone Therapy Levels II and III, which focus on deeper emotional and psychic aspects and connect us to universal consciousness. Here we explore the possibility of the human energy fields extending to an even higher spiritual level known as the *causal body* or *field;* this can be considered the closest thing to the soul. The practitioner will then be ready to explore the more advanced techniques.

As we embark on this journey to align with the cosmic forces that flow throughout our bodies and the universe and to enhance our health and well-being, we elevate ourselves into a higher state of being. Yet when we understand that our sense of identity is in constant flux, we can allow ourselves to be more authentic in our spiritual development. At this level, miracles can occur.

* * *

When I dream, it is just a dream.

When we all have the same dream,

it is the beginning of a new reality.

* * *

Many people strive for serenity, balance and physical wellness in this fast-paced world. I have developed the Stone Therapy Balancing Treatment in response to this quest. The integration of Stone Therapy Massage and Chakra Balancing dissolves stress, removes blockages and neutralizes negative energies, inducing a feeling of well-being and balance. Taking us internally, it helps us to rediscover our vital energy, our highest level of being.

Stone Therapy is a fusion, a blend of Eastern and Western philosophies. It has been intergraded as an ancient method with modern viewpoints, producing an entirely new approach. Join me now in discovering the newly developed Stone Therapy.

FOREWORD

In ancient days, the healing art of Stone Therapy was designed specifically to enhance physical and spiritual balancing. This book, in having found its way to you, is itself a link. Some of the stone application information shared within this book is very ancient and has been passed on from family member to family member through generations.

As we begin to reawaken, examine and modify ancient traditions, we will discover that all primitive cultures had a natural evolutionary development from a biological origin. Man created his primitive beliefs based on fear. By means of his illusions and delusions, these beliefs evolved beyond nature worship, and Man began to acquire the roots of spirituality, always conditioned by social environment.

Primitive man feared and worshiped manifestations of nature's powerful forces such as earthquakes, volcanoes, storms and floods. These inexplicable phenomena were once termed "acts of God," and in many regions of the world, they are still worshiped as icons today.

With its characteristic durability and permanence, stone is in many cultures a symbol of divine power, with its ability to produce fire from the sparks produced by striking two stones together. Since the early stages of humanity, stones were used to make tools and weapons. Our ancient ancestors were quite frequently able to differentiate between stones of various mineralogy, and thus their quality.

Initially, objects of worship were stones that impressed early Man by their sudden appearance in a cultivated field due to natural but unobserved occurrences. References to sacred stones are numerous in ancient texts. In fact, many of the Old Testament psalms were inscribed on stone. The

Bible refers to Jacob sleeping on a stone and even anointing it.

In the Middle East, a stone was a sign of God and was covered with libations (pouring out of wine in honor) or anointed with oil.

The significance of stone blocks that were formed naturally rather than by human hands had strong spiritual significance as expressed in Exodus 20:25: "and if thou wilt, make it of hewn [smoothed or shaped], for if thou lift up thy tool upon it, thou has polluted it." Twelve precious stones adorned the breastplate of the Jewish high priest: agate, amethyst, beryl, carnelian, jasper, jacinth, lapis lazuli, nephrite, ruby, tarsis and peridot. The names of the twelve tribes of Israel were to be engraved, one on each stone.

Almost all Arabian tribes paid respect to a specific black stone known as the Kaaba, located in a temple at Mecca. What Yahweh was to the Jews, the Kaaba stone was to the Arabs.

Ayurveda, India's ancient healing system, has its own history of specific stones, some semi-precious, which are used to balance planetary influences and to act on life forces. Ayurveda also uses oxidized and purified stones in medicine, including individual stones to influence the doshas (physical energies). The Ayurvedic system believes, for example, that agate decreases Kapha (the dosha for body structure) and assists in spiritual awakening and protection from fear. Amethyst is believed to decrease Vata (the dosha for body movement) and Pitta (the dosha for metabolism) to balance the emotions and promote a sense of compassion and hope.

Some tribes in India still view specific stones as sacred. For example, the uniqueness of Nepal's Z stone is in its abstract patterns of circles and lines. It is considered a stone of protection for those who wear or hold it. The more circles (eyes) the stone has, the more valuable it is said to be.

All ancient clans and tribes had their sacred stones and rituals, including the indigenous tribes of Mexico. The Aztecs and the Roramuni (meaning *today the people*) were kept true to their ancient customs by a combination of wilderness homeland, an inherent value system of obligation to fellow man, and a devotion to ancient ways. The exact origin of their traditional sweat lodges is unclear, but it is believed the tradition began with the Olmecs around 1200-10000 B.C. in Mesoamerica's initial culture. Later the ancients brought into Christianity long-established rituals and symbols, replacing things of a contemplative nature. They preferred to pray, however, in a ritual manner such as in the *temazcal,* a manmade clay or stone hut.

The word *temazcal* originates from Nahualt, the founder of the Aztec empire's language, and means *bathhouse.* There are said to be remains of temazcals in some old Mayan ruins as well.

The temazcal is part of a worldwide tradition of steam bath similar to the Turkish and Finnish sauna, from people who believed that body and mind were inseparable, from a time when God and nature were entwined. To enter the temazcal, one was covered in volcanic mud and then rinsed before entering on bended knees in prayer. Once everyone was inside the hut, special lava stones were placed in a central pit, and water that was infused with herbs such as sage or rosemary was thrown on the stones to repel negative energy.

Amber-colored stones were also used in this ritual. These are not crystals but are formed from solidified tree resin. Amber is believed to promote wisdom and altruism, and is a useful healer. Prayers were in the form of dance rather than the spoken word.

The basic temazcal ritual practiced in modern day has not changed much from its ancient origins. Each of the temazcaleros who conducts this ritual, however, has his own individual method.

Sometimes groups of stones were used in ceremonies. The Greeks used a cluster of thirty. Romans believed in throwing a stone in the air whenever invoking the planet Mercury.

The Ancients also held a reverence for specific stones in various shapes. Porous stones such as the Chinese Bian stone 2000 years ago were said to contain curative properties. Even now, most modern cultures manifest a curious degree of longing for specific types of stones such as jewels.

In ancient Mexico, turquoise (in Aztec, xihuitl) was one of the most admired gemstones; only jade was more valued. Sky blue turquoise symbolized heavenly and earthly forces.

* * *

Chapter 1

THE JOURNEY

Greetings.

It has been said that everyone has a story.

I have dedicated a majority of my life to the understanding and practice of Massage and Energy Therapy and to a holistic approach to all things.

During the past thirty years or so, each time I had a new insight or worked my way through another challenge, I would say, "Someday I am going to write a book." And on a deeper level, I knew that someday I would. So here I find myself with a deep sense of purpose and gratitude to the many friends and peers who planted the seed and urged me to write this book.

Time was my most frequently used excuse for delay: "Oh, I am too busy. I have a workshop to facilitate, another video to produce, a new manual to write." The true catalyst was actually seeing a Web site that duplicated mine almost word for word. Then I knew it was time.

According to the Massage Association, we were a $4 billion industry in 2003. It has taken us years of working hard, improving our standards and lobbying to bring Massage Therapy to this level.

Try to imagine what it was like in Mid-America in 1972 when I became a therapist. Massage was not popular as it is today. It was primarily available in YMCAs or private clubs and was dominated mostly by (male) masseurs. The few (female) masseuses were perceived as strong, burly and Swedish. The other options, massage parlors, were illegal, so not really an option. The early massage therapists accepted their role in educating communities and clients about the benefits of massage. We were the early pioneers of our industry.

Now that we have reached a higher level of acceptance and popularity, let us not backtrack by offering unprofessional services using Crock-Pots, electric skillets and labeled turkey roasters in conjunction with our Stone Therapy services.

In this still maturing industry, I am keenly aware of the issues facing our practitioners, and one of the most problematic is misinformation. As the market has rapidly expanded, especially on a global level, people have noticed the effectiveness of this new concept, and the marketplace is becoming increasingly competitive. Consequently, inaccurate information regarding the actual therapy, its application and related products has begun to appear, along with inconsistencies from so-called "experts" sharing their speculative interpretations.

Opinions are the cheapest commodity on Earth. Some of this information is firmly contraindicative and so easily discernable as achieving new depths of human absurdity and a cause of confusion in our industry, especially as far as its adaptations and product use are concerned.

It has been extremely disturbing to observe this trend. Although I have been aware of the need for me to act, frankly, at first I did not quite know how. When I shared these concerns with my peers and other leaders in the Industry, the response was always the same: "Sonia, you can influence the outcome. You are the world's foremost authority on Stone Therapy. Why don't you write a book?" I have taken this advice, and after three years in the process, I can tell you I have tremendous respect for anyone with published work.

I receive daily e-mail requests from all over the world for current information on the subject of Stone Massage. I have always been aware of the tremendous need for accurate information, because of the sheer newness of the method and because there is so little factual information published. I feel a responsibility to share my knowledge. My hope is that this book will provide you with new insights concerning Stone Therapy as a safe, effective alternative and a complimentary modality to your current massage practice. It is my life's work.

I hope my story inspires you to dream and to persist in your personal search. Find your heart's longing, find your passion, live life fully. As Oriah Mountain Dreamer has said so beautifully, "What if the question is not 'why am I so infrequently the person I really want to be,' but 'why do I so infrequently want to be the person I really am?'" Never, ever give up hope.

* * *

This book is dedicated to all committed non-invasive body workers who, through their professionalism, idealism and love of their chosen vocation, produce profound, positive change on so many levels. You are the primary reason I am sharing this information with the world.

* * *

Chapter 2

MY STONE JOURNEY

The time was the mid-1950s. The Valka camp in Nuremberg, Germany was a dismal refugee camp for displaced persons. My mother, German-born Christine Schmitz, lost her first husband at the beginning of World War II when she was only twenty-one years old. A few years later, she lost her German citizenship when she married a Hungarian who eventually left her desolate and struggling to survive.

The Valka camp was our home. We were refugees in our own country. My mother felt hopeless with three young children to care for. My brother, Teno, was then only a few months old. My younger sister, Sylvia, was four years old with raven black hair and hazel eyes like my mother had. I was just one year older with long, golden locks like wheat and sparkling brown eyes.

I recall one particular night quite vividly, the night that changed my life forever. My world was a one-room barrack inside this refugee camp. It was the middle of winter and so cold outside that I could see frost formed thickly all around the window. Occasionally I could catch a glimpse of falling snowflakes. I could hear the howling wind blowing against the frail wood walls, our meager protection from the exterior world.

Although the room was dimly lit, I remember the permeating warmth from the wood burner in the corner. Even today, it still gives me a strange sense of comfort when I transport myself back to that moment, somehow frozen in time in my mind.

I recall my sister, Sylvia, and I sitting on a blanket on the wooden floor. We were going on a trip. We watched our mother prepare the small satchels that she had hand-crocheted, filling them with fruit for our long journey. I remember being excited about our adventure, so innocently unaware that this trip would separate me from my family for the next seven years.

We were so poor that my mother had contacted a humanitarian agency who placed needy children with foster families. What is unimaginable yet true is that they sent us to another country. We boarded a train headed for Belgium, just Sylvia and I, just four and five years old. Worse yet, we spoke only German and Belgians spoke French. My initial excitement turned to concern before long. I missed our mother, although as long as Sylvia was with me, I thought everything would be all right.

Eventually, we were awakened by the jolt of the train coming to a stop when it arrived at Embourg, a suburb of Liege, Belgium. I grasped Sylvia's hand and we stepped off the train in a strange, new country.

A representative was there to greet us from Catholic Charities, which was placing persons like us in private homes. Two families were also there, one for Sylvia and one for me. The realization that we were to be separated was so traumatic that I cried, kicked and screamed. The foster family that was assigned to care for Sylvia was suddenly reassigned to me because they claimed to speak a little German. This claim turned out not to be true.

I was a very frightened little girl, separated from both my mother and sister and going off to live with complete strangers who could not speak my language. These foster parents were in their sixties and had never had children of their own, so they had no idea how to deal with me, how to comfort me or how to communicate until I could learn French.

I was terrified as we approached the villa that would be my home for the next seven years. My foster parents, who I learned to call Uncle George and Auntie Maggy, could not stop my hysterical cries that entire day and night. Auntie Maggy would often recount later how she had cradled me in her lap until the next morning. I was heartbroken.

I received an excellent education at Les Pensionnat du Sacre Coeur, a private Catholic all-girl school, but the nuns were disciplinarians to the worst degree. Although I was naturally left-handed, I was slapped with the ruler every day until I learned to use my right hand.

All my clothes were handmade and I wanted for nothing material, but what I longed for was love and acceptance. My foster parents were both very unstable and at times even emotionally and physically abusive towards me.

Uncle George died when I was eight years old, but not before his severe symptoms of Alzheimer's disease and bouts of abuse toward me and toward his wife caused me additional trauma. I recall actually fearing for our lives during this very dark period. I remember my relief when

George died and I realized he would no longer be able to terrorize us.

After Uncle George was gone, though, Auntie Maggy isolated me from the world. Other than school and very rare trips to the city, we lived a very secluded life. I was all she had.

My life was confusing, sad and lonely. Prayer helped me to cope with the pain and emptiness in my heart. As that little girl, I prayed diligently to God and to the Virgin Mary. A small statue of Mary on the stand beside my bed gave off the most beautiful luminous glow at night and made me feel safe. My faith has never wavered to this day. Through faith, I believe all things are possible.

When I was about seven or eight years old, a neighbor suffered a stroke and his entire left side became paralyzed. A masseur came by frequently to administer therapy until eventually the neighbor recovered. This event had a tremendous impact on me at my young age. I knew from that time on that when I grew up, I needed to become a massage therapist. I wanted to help people feel better.

When I was twelve, my mother came to Embourg to take me home to Germany. Although this should have been the answer to my dreams, it felt very strange to see her after seven years. The train ride back to Erlangen was a long, silent one because I could no longer speak German and we were unable to communicate with each other. Ironically, I was in the same situation leaving Belgium as when I had arrived seven years earlier.

Back in Germany, I had to relearn my native language, attempt to reconnect with my mother and siblings and fit in at school. This time was a nightmare for me. Before long, I was diagnosed with a severe ulcer and spent some time healing in the hospital.

A year later, I was beginning to settle in at school and make new friends when my mother made another life-changing decision: to emigrate to the United States. She longed for a better life for all of us. So we packed our few belongings and came to what I deem to be the greatest country in the world. At thirteen years old, my life became extremely challenging once again.

Mother enrolled us in a Catholic school, although we could not speak a word of English. This was the 1960s, so we were left to our own devices to learn the language. Other kids taunted us and we would often return from school in tears, vowing never to speak German again. Regrettably, that is exactly what we did: we lost our native language.

Our little family settled in Portsmouth, Ohio. My dream to become a masseuse kept me going all this time. The only accredited massage school nearby at that time was the College of Masso/ Therapy on East Gay Street in Columbus, Ohio. The year was 1972.

When I met with Mrs. Thompson, the school's owner, she frankly tried to discourage me from becoming a massage therapist. In retrospect, I cannot blame her; I was young and weighed barely 100 pounds. But I was on a mission and would not take "no" for an answer. As mentioned here earlier, when I started in this field, legal massage establishments were mostly YMCAs and if a masseuse was even on staff, she was thought to be burly and Swedish. But I was determined.

Mrs. Thompson began by asking me questions to determine my character, and then offered me a first-hand experience of a massage and reflexology treatment. When she applied pressure to the uterus reflex point in my foot, I experienced tremendous pain. This is the area located below the medial maleolus of the tibia, also referred to as the interior ankle area. Mrs. Thompson suggested I consult with my medical doctor, as did my mother, who was by then a Registered Nurse (R.N.) at nearby Mercy Hospital. By then other symptoms had appeared: extreme weight loss, fatigue, etc.

I was diagnosed with Grade V cervical cancer detected in the early stages. I recall the doctor's concern as to the prognosis: since it required curettage on my cervix, there was a possibility I would never be able to bear children.

I proceeded with the surgery, feeling lonely and frightened. The next morning in the recovery room, I was awakened by a rustling sound and looked up to see a priest standing over me, holding a gleaming gold chalice in his hands. I had not requested communion and had not had a chance to go to confession before surgery, with so much on my mind. In my grogginess, I tried to decline, but the priest insisted and very quickly was gone. I didn't give the incident much thought again until I began writing this book.

The reflexology procedure performed on me by Mrs. Thompson at her school that day was the catalyst that led to the discovery of my cancer. Life for me would never ever be the same again.

In time, I recovered, married and experienced another miracle: the birth of my son, Alex. As I began at last to live a normal life, I knew that I had been given a tremendous gift. I was on the correct path and my mission was real. All the suffering I had endured had not only strengthened me, but also taught me to allow myself to be guided. I knew that massage therapy was the vehicle for me to demonstrate tremendous compassion, empathy and love toward my fellow man through the power of human touch. And so began this Stone Journey.

I graduated from massage school and sat for the exam. In 1972, accreditation was given by a division of the State Medical Board through a two-day testing process. On the first day was a written exam and on the next, hands-on demonstrations with questions. The process has certainly changed since then.

After passing my boards, my true journey began and I absorbed all the knowledge I could: Japanese and Chinese massage, energy work, philosophy, reflexology and its applications, acupuncture and its meridian systems, Reiki, Polarity, all adaptations in both eastern and western philosophies and their effects on the body's natural healing process. I have spent many years perfecting my craft. During my learning process, my appetite for knowledge and thorough understanding was insatiable. Always searching for a balance, I gradually incorporated all these new insights into my massage practice. I believe that when we open our hearts and minds, a tremendous shift can occur in this atmosphere, bringing forth significant events.

My zealous interest in and application of stones in conjunction with my massage practice began many years ago with a desire for crystals and their many forms: raw, quartz, pendulums, pyramids and so on.

I was completely unaware then but am now perfectly convinced that crystals, stones and semi-precious stones actually choose us if we are receptive to the process. This is why at times we are so attracted and drawn to specific stones. I believe they emit minute electrical impulses very similar to our body's own frequency.

Once the contact has been made, a crystal can attract and repel. If it is meant for you, it will find its way to you. When its benefit to you has ended, it will pass to someone else. When your journey with it has ended, you will give it away, lose it or perhaps just place it in a drawer.

Since the 1970s, friends and colleagues who have observed my enthusiasm have brought me semi-precious stones from their travels, sparking my interest in a new world of minerals. I have spent many years experimenting with specific subtle vibrational resonances that these stones seem to emit and the correlation when applied to specific points on the body, including massage. These were my first clues to vibrational healing.

In 1979, I realized another dream when I opened the doors to my first holistic day spa, offering all aspects of the holistic concept: acupuncture, European facials, reflexology, massage, aromatherapy, and natural hair and nail care. During those early days, I once requested that my staff pre-soak a client's feet in a green tea footbath prior to a pedicure. They came to me horrified when the tea mixture stained the client's feet. Although we can laugh about it now, it was not very amusing at the time.

In the early 1970s in Southern Ohio, I heard raves about an elderly gentleman who practiced herbology and irology. Since my herb guru was Adele Davis and my favorite book was *Sugar Blues* by Gloria Swanson, I was fascinated and made an appointment.

Chief, as everyone called him, was a descendant of the Shawnee Indian tribe that settled hundreds of years ago in the Ohio Valley. Chief was the first person who actually placed a warm stone in my hand as an integral part of treatment. I was amazed. He shared with me how the Ancients used stones for grounding and in their sweat lodges.

The Shawnee Indians' spirituality profoundly resonated their tremendous respect for Mother Earth and their understanding of the stones' connection to the Earth, millions of years old. Chief explained that one reason the Indians wore moccasins was to walk the Earth softly.

Thus began my long road of trial and discovery with the stones. Some of my initial findings seemed to indicate that Stone Therapy could elicit a relaxation response that involves restorative functions of the body and deactivates the stress response. Benefits include soothing frazzled nerves, easing muscle tension, restoring muscle fatigue and promoting energy balancing and well-being. As the shift occurs, the undercurrent of stress dissipates and energy can again flow freely.

In specific stone practice, it seems we are experiencing the directing of core energy. I sense a certain gentle, elegant energy pulse encircling the recipient and the practitioner—*cradling* us is really the only way I can describe it.

Our bodies are made up of colossal energy fields. They function best by moving along and clearing the interactive, stagnant field of energy debris caused primarily by physical and emotional trauma disguised in many forms. This clearing and restorative balance is achieved through a combination of very specific massage techniques, stones and vibrational techniques. When proper function and balance are restored, our vital energy can flow freely once again.

I believe this process to be a catalyst to optimum health. In my opinion, no other therapy induces such a deep state of relaxation and produces such profound change on so many levels. My conviction comes also from a very specific discovery concerning my stone work with cancer patients.

According to the American Cancer Society, more than 1.2 million Americans were diagnosed with cancer in 2002. No single therapeutic agent can be compared in healing to the touch of the human hand and a warm stone, creating a conduit to help patients reconnect with themselves.

Stone massage is one of the fastest growing and most frequently requested treatments, according to spa industry experts. It is now available in most spas, salons, resorts, and in a seemingly unlikely environment, a few hospital oncology departments. While it would be absurd to suggest stone massage as a cure for cancer, research has shown that a variety of touch methods positively affect many ill effects from radiation treatment and cancer itself including fatigue, nausea, edema, pain and insomnia.

Before I sold all my other business ventures to devote myself solely to the development of Stone Therapy, the last day spa I owned was in Hollywood, Florida. Desiring to offer my services to cancer patients in the community, I contacted the American Cancer Society. Through their "Look Good, Feel Good" program at Memorial Hospital, my staff and I were thoroughly trained by the Cancer Society and hospital staff. Every month, eight to ten patients receiving radiation or chemotherapy were directed to my day spa, where we would fit them with wigs and apply makeup provided by the Cancer Society.

I also personally volunteered my services on a therapeutic level. Cancer patients reported to me how gentle massage with the stones decreased their anxiety and sense of isolation, improved their mood, and lessened their overall psychological distress.

Cancer weakens our hope and slowly separates our body and soul, but stone massage is a source of calming, soothing, nurturing—a gentle, loving touch. At present, I am aware of only one facility offering an oncology massage program: the Sherer Institute in Santa Fe, New Mexico.

On this subject, I highly recommend Gayle MacDonald's book, *Medicine Hands*. But I always add this caution: Any treatment of cancer patients must be administered under the supervision and care of the accompanying oncology physician as well as a specially trained therapist.

As I was nearing my twentieth year in the spa industry, I felt it was time for a new journey. I sold my day spas and decided to take a break for the first time since I was sixteen. I had been divorced for ten years and there was nowhere that I had to be.

Since I lived near the ocean, I spent the first month or so pondering the next phase of my life from the beach through meditation, yoga and a lot of thought.

One day I came across a flier from a holistic lifestyle center announcing a new class to help individuals determine what they should truly be doing on their life journey – how to find their life's passion. I made an appointment the next day and met Lera, a gentle soul who asked the appropriate questions to become a vehicle to my uncovering my Stone Journey. Little did I suspect that day that my life was about to change again, and drastically.

During this period, I also met a new boyfriend, Marcel, who was very intrigued by my work and by how I spoke of the benefits of the stones. Since he came from the industrial spectrum, this was a new world for him. Periodically he would inquire, "DO YOU REALLY BELIEVE in this? Can they really make a difference?" Each time, my response was to share with him, with intense love, belief and reason, my passion and my vision. This went on for several months.

I envisioned this concept being used in health spas and related industries worldwide and on the Internet. Remembering that there was nothing about Stone Therapy on the Internet, I could imagine it in specialty shops everywhere, not only for massage but also for facials, manicures, pedicures, and *thallaso* treatments (water therapy) at exclusive wellness facilities.

Marcel would chuckle at my vision and say, "Whoa! Not so fast!" But a few months later, again he would ask and again I would share my beliefs and dreams about Stone Therapy. Finally, one day my response was so poignant that Marcel said, "Let's do it."

Initially, we tested the market by sending fliers to therapists promoting the concept of Stone

Therapy and accompanying education, and the response was overwhelmingly, "Yes, yes, yes." Since then, our pace has been non-stop: 700 seminars worldwide, five instructional videos and DVDs, instruction manuals and a book.

A million stones or so later, while Marcel is no longer my boyfriend, he remains my business partner. The stage has been set. My dream of sharing the power of healing touch as a catalyst for change has become a reality. Presently we are the #1 leading company in the world, with our primary focus of stone distribution and related education continuing with a worldwide network.

* * *

Chapter 3

ANCIENT STONES

Gateway to Health and Harmony

Stone Therapy: Let us begin by exploring its origin. Various unique forms and adaptations of Stone Therapy have been part of the Eastern world's regime of science for thousands of years. Healers from every corner of the globe have incorporated stones in one form or another.

Many cultures recognize the role played by energy release. Using warm stones that are formed by sedimentary and volcanic action, Stone Therapy is effective for two primary reasons: the stone's thermal conduction effect causes local and systematic changes in the body, and it influences the energy centers of both body and mind, causing a transformation on a multitude of levels.

We are reminded that we are presently in a resurgence of the timeless interest in stones. Gems certainly possess a unique power of attraction, filled as they are with the file of life while adorning our bodies and soothing our souls. Philosophers speak of the stark contrast between ephemeral humanity and the indestructible rock, gem or fossil. Gems and minerals have always been perceived as bones of Mother Earth. People also love to collect and wear choice specimens.

Through the ages, many kinds of stones have served as amulets, treasures and charms, including quartz crystal (silicon dioxide), which is only one of many silicates. All stones contain some amount of silicon dioxide, or quartz. In addition to their shapes, colors and beauty, the timeless attraction is also an aesthetic response.

Many traditions and myths point to Man's long established rituals of worshipping certain stones and divine spirits. Icelanders, for instance, revered a stone known as the Mother of Prosperity.

Certain African tribes believed that stones with holes in them symbolized birth and the womb. In yet other cultures, midwives rotated certain stones above a woman in childbirth while whistling to insure safe passage for the newborn. Patriarchal societies showed great hostility toward ancient stone figures.

In Brittany, many prehistoric domens (two large upright stones set with a space in-between and capped by a horizontal stone) were known as "hot stones." They were believed to transfer their powers to infertile women who sat on them, their heat symbolizing life force. The stones were believed to store up energy and pass it along to those who came into contact with them. These interpretations document how deeply rooted our beliefs and associations with stones are.

The Stone of Sconce

Originally associated with the crowning of Scottish kings, the famous Stone of Sconce was moved to England in 1296. Its place under the Coronation Chair in London's Westminster Abbey symbolizes the rule of English monarchs over Scotland. The superstitious once said it was a hag, or fairy grandmother, which was turned to stone when cursed by a Christian missionary.

Popular interest in minerals is not only for their qualities of color, density, solidity, relative indestructibility and scientific curiosity. Today there are once again more esoteric reasons as they symbolize the universality and inseparability of matter even among the multitudes of diverse forms. We are all connected.

Stone Therapy is one of the most ancient ways of health maintenance and treatment, sometimes referred to as the "Stone remedy." Stone

Therapy was highly valued as one of the earliest treatment methods used by healers in China. Classic writings on Chinese medicine show how massage methods flourished during that era. The Zhou dynasty in 700 B.C., for example, referred to massage as *anwu,* a combination of massage, specific stones and acupuncture.

Many indigenous medical systems in different parts of the world correspond to China's experience. It was presented in much the very same way by Indian physicians in their books of Yajurvedic medicine and by the Hippocratic physicians of Greece.

The connection between crystal stones and the human body has been known for thousands of years. In Traditional Chinese Medicine (TCM), it goes back 5,000 years and is still in use today. TCM used crystals as part of its pharmacopoeia with a strong understanding of their applications.

The three legendary emperors – Fu His, Shen Nung and Huang Ti – are considered the founders of the art of healing. The first record of Stone Therapy is in the ancient Chinese text of *Huang Ti*, known in its translation as the *Yellow Emperor*. Research on this text is still incomplete, but scholars estimate its inception at 2597 to 2577 B.C., over 4,000 years ago.

This text describes the use of breathing exercises, massage and special stones, as well as *moxibustion*, a medical practice that later spread to Japan and other Asian countries. Moxibustion, or moxa treatment, is performed by burning small cones of dried leaves on certain designated points of the body, generally the same points as those used in acupuncture. While there were few texts on anatomy and surgery, the ancient writings on internal diseases are voluminous.

The *Nei Ching* text about 200 A.D. included massage, herb and stone applications and suggestions for their use. These are especially prominent in the subtext of *Su Wen*, written from early conversations between the Emperor and his physician.

In most Asiatic countries, scientific medicine has not permeated very deeply. The lack of facilities and practitioners made a decent income in this field impossible in rural areas. The foreignness of scientific medicine to the majority of the population contributes to most Asians not receiving medical care from trained physicians, but instead from indigenous practitioners following pre-set ways of the ancients or medieval medicine. They feel the pulse, examine the patient, reason their symptoms and treat as their ancestors did many centuries ago.

After the East Han Dynasty (206 B.C. to 25 A.D.), the Chinese combined Stone Therapy with *meridians* and collaterals therapy. After that, it disappeared from history records, due primarily to poorly preserved heritage and the shortage of suitable material, exemplified only by the scraping method (Guasha) and other sparsely used stone such as water ox. Dr. Wang Ping, a distinguished scholar in the Tang dynasty (762 A.D.) remarked, "There was special stone for treating disease in ancient age, but this technique has vanished now."

The use of Stone Therapy lessened and acupuncture flourished, possibly due in part to the popularity of fine and exquisite things symbolized by therapeutic needles. Both Stone Therapy and acupuncture share the theory of meridians and collaterals (Jingluo bodily channels in TCM conceptions); the difference lies in using concrete manipulation.

Papyrus Ebers (1150 B.C.), one of the most ancient Egyptian medical treaties, also refers to the twelve meridians. The bone etchings of ancient Eskimos suggest they used simple acupressure with stones applied mainly at congested or painful areas. This practice corresponds to the simplest form of acupuncture in which only the *locus dolenti* and not the distant part is stimulated. This method is applied to tender areas that dissipate as treatment corrects imbalances in the body.

The Bantus of South Africa were known to scratch certain parts of the body with specific mineral stones and herbs to help cure disease, methods primarily administered by the tribe's medicine man.

* * *

Chapter 4

ANCIENT STONE THERAPY

The Chinese Bian Stone

The system of Bian Stone, as Stone Therapy was originally known, is one of the most ancient methods of health maintenance and treatment and the mother of acupuncture and moxibustion. This method was recorded as a separate medical system in *Yellow Emperor's Classic*.

Traditional Chinese Medicine (TCM) includes not only Bian Stone Therapy but also acupuncture, moxibustion, physical and breathing exercise (Daoyin), Tuina (Chinese Massage) and Chinese herb medication. Until 1985, the Chinese Acupuncture-moxibustion Society was a branch of the China National TCM Society.

When Bian Stone Therapy was originally developed, it was combined with knowledge on meridians and collaterals. In *Bo Book*, an ancient book recording bodily channels, Bian Stone manipulations in medical practice were described in detail, indicating that this application is as old as meridians and collaterals therapy.

As mentioned earlier, Bian Stone Therapy was an important component of TCM but gradually faded when the Chinese ceased to hand it down, until it seemed to disappear entirely in and around the Han Dynasty.

In recent years, thanks to the efforts of distinguished geologists and scholars of TCM, the source of this essential therapeutic tool was restored at last when they determined Sibin Floating Stone to be the most excellent material for producing Bian Stone.

Continuing extensive research has developed into the New Bian Stone Therapy with a series of special applications. Additional research on meridians and collaterals, such as combining them with new manipulations, has led to a new stage of science and awareness. In combination with the research obtained in archaeology, the ancient technique has been revived. Researchers have also made considerable investigation into massive TCM documents.

Experimentation and practice have proven the salutary properties of this and other stones in promoting human health. For example, a stone therapist can work on the entire meridians (a conception of bodily channels in TCM) rather than a few acu-points for a more thorough unblocking of channels. Easing both pain and anxiety is the strong point of this therapy, yet it maintains the flavor of the ancient ways.

* * *

The Sibin Floating Stone

Numerous archaeological findings and cures by the unique Sibin Floating Stone found along China's Si River led to its choice as the updated Bian Stone.

The new systematic Bian Stone therapeutic method results from scientific tests on Sibin Floating Stone by five authoritative scientific institutes. Through considerable clinical practice and geological testing, Sibin Stone has been proven remarkably effective in the treatment of disease and in health preservation. Research has found, for example, that wearing a small Bian pendant on the chest can help a patient with heart disease to restore normal cardiac rhythm.

Chemical Analysis

The effectiveness of a specific stone in treating disharmony in the human body is largely dependent on the stone's properties. According to the Geologist Test Center of the National Nuclear Industry, calcium carbonate is the major ingredient – over fifty percent – in Sibin Floating Stone. Other key concentrations include calcium, iron, phosphorus, potassium and sodium. More than thirty salutary trace elements found include chromium, magnesium, zinc and strontium.

No toxins were discovered in Sibin Floating Stone. In fact, the stone's radiation was found to be much lower than that of a normal stone, so there is no risk of harm to the body. These results were presented by the Institute of Geology of Academic Sinica in Taiwan.

When the Guiyang Geochemistry Institute of the China Academy of Sciences in Guiyang, Guizhao, China did micro-sectioning tests on this stone, the major mineral revealed was micro crystal calcite. Each unit of the particle is less than 0.03 mm, far lower than the structural units of other rocks. This property makes this stone unique when rubbed on the skin. It is historically a widely applied treatment in Chinese medicine, based almost entirely upon a complicated method of palpitation coupled with observation for external changes.

* * *

Ultrasonic Tests

The ultrasonic features of Sibin Floating Stone were tested by the State Seismology Bureau of China. When struck, this stone can produce not only sound, but also considerable ultrasonic wave pulses with frequencies from 20 to 2,000 KHz. When rubbed against the body, rich ultrasonic wave pulses can improve microcirculation, reduce redundant fat and inhibit the growth of tumors. In terms of TCM, the process means clearing bodily channels of evil *qi*, expelling toxin and eliminating excessive heat.

* * *

Below is a comparison of Sibin Stone to various other materials for making a therapeutic plate. It shows the number of ultrasonic wave pulses and the frequency range when the materials are scraped against the back of a human hand.

Material	Pulses	Range (KHz)
Blue Jade	20-800	1938
Horn of Water Ox	20-200	353
Sheep Grease Jade	20-1000	2249
Wood Fish Stone	20-1000	2480
Sibin Floating Stone	20-2000	3698

The advantages of Sibin Stone are obvious, especially when compared with Horn of Water Ox, which is the normal cutaneous scraping plate.

Thermal Effects

To discover how the human body is influenced by the application of Sibin Stone, infrared remote sensing tests were performed by the Institute of Remote Sensing at Academia Sinica. Subjects were selected whose demeanor was calm physically and emotionally in a testing situation.

Infrared thermal images of each subject's face or hand were recorded for five minutes to ensure the image was stable. Then a piece of Sibin Floating Stone was placed about 5 cm from the skin. After thirty minutes, an increase in temperature at the site was recorded of 0.5 to 2 degrees, depending on the subject.

Infrared Radiation Spectrum Tests

The average peak range of infrared radiation in rocks should be attributed to the testing wavelength's variation of 8 to 11 um. Once the testing wavelength exceeds 12 um, the radiation decreases drastically. However, the range of infrared radiation of Sibin Stone remained high when the testing wavelength varied from 8 to 14.5 um. Note that 14.5 um is the upper limit of the most advanced machine for measuring infrared spectral radiation. This indicates that the stone's infrared radiation spectrum can extend beyond 16 um, which is extremely wide. This wide range and other unique qualities of Sibin Floating Stone make it the superior choice for Bian Stone Therapy.

The knowledge of using different types of stones for therapeutic purposes as handed down from ancient times has experienced a recent resurgence in China.

Chapter 5

UNDERSTANDING
MINERALS AND STONES

There is something so wonderful about stones. They are invaluable for the many ways in which they serve us. If we understand the importance of our Earth and the stones beneath our feet, then we understand Earth and Man are inseparable.

Chemical elements are the building blocks of all materials including rocks, which are elements or compounds found naturally in the Earth's crust. Some rocks are fixed chemical compositions, while others are a series of related compounds in which one metallic element may replace another in whole or part. This explains differences in color and other physical properties.

Today, hundreds of elements are known, but only a dozen or so were known in ancient times. The most recent finds were during atom-splitting experiments.

The Earth can be viewed as a gigantic chemical factory, wherein all the chemical elements are mixed and combined. Minerals are naturally occurring chemical compounds and elements. There are about 2,400 mineral species that have been identified as "rock forming," and approximately 100 of these are routinely cut into gemstones. A rock is made up of one or more minerals, each chemically different from the others.

Molten magna, or lava, is generated by molten currents of minerals flowing from the core of our planet up through volcanoes. As lava cools down, it becomes volcanic stone with a permanent imprint of the magnetic energy of its geomagnetic field.

There are three groups of natural rock: igneous, sedimentary and metamorphic.

1. *IGNEOUS* rocks are formed at high temperatures from molten materials.

2. *SEDIMENTARY* rocks are formed by the action of water, wind or organic agents.

3. *METAMORPHIC* rocks have been altered by heat, pressure or chemical action.

Igneous rocks comprise about ninety-five percent of the Earth's crust. Heat or pressure causes localized melting of the deep crust and mantle rock within the Earth, creating bodies of molten rock called magmas. These fire-formed rocks are of two main types: intrusive and extrusive.

Intrusive rocks, such as granite, cool gradually deep within the Earth. As magma cools slowly, minerals have time to crystallize. Granite, for example, is famous for its beauty, strength and durability, containing crystals of quartz and feldspar in addition to other minerals. Due to its mixture of minerals, granite is usually spotted but can also present itself in white, pink, gray or red.

Extrusive rocks, such as basalt, form when magma erupts to cool rapidly at the Earth's surface as a hardened flow of lava. Colors vary from black, dark gray or purple to a greenish tint. These spectacular volcanic stones are rich in magnesium and/or ferrous iron.

Intrusive and extrusive rock may form from the same magma and be identical in composition but differ in texture if they cool at different rates. Thus, extrusive rocks tend to be coarse and intrusive rocks, finely grained.

Sedimentary rocks cover about three-fourths of the Earth's surface and are extremely varied in texture, composition and color. Nearly all are made of materials that have been moved from a place of origin to a new place, which can be a distance of only a few feet or thousands of miles. Currents, wind, waves, running water, ice and gravity move materials on the Earth's surface by action that takes place on or very near the surface over millions of years.

Weathering is the process by which rocks are broken down by the atmosphere and other factors in the environment. There are two types of weathering: *mechanical* and *chemical.*

Mechanical weathering is a breakdown of rock into smaller pieces with no chemical composition. The major agents in mechanical weathering are temperature changes, frost action, plant roots and flaking.

Chemical weathering is a breakdown of rock in which a chemical reaction occurs, caused by at least one of the following reactions:

Oxygen: In the presence of vapor, oxygen from the air combines with the iron found in many rocks to oxidize. The rust produced by oxidation crumbles away easily, causing the rocks to fall apart.

1. Acid:

(a) Protists such as lichen that grows on rocks and bacteria that decay produce acids that slowly dissolve some materials in rocks.

(b) When carbon dioxide in the atmosphere dissolves in water, it produces a weak acid. When water containing this acid flows over limestone, the limestone dissolves and is carried away by the water. In this manner, limestone caves are formed, such as Mammoth Cave in Kentucky.

Sandstone is the second most common sedimentary rock and consists of particles that have been worn from pre-existing rocks and then deposited on sea or riverbeds. The color may be red, brown, gray, green or yellow. The Grand Canyon is a dramatic display of this stone.

Another sedimentary rock, soft coal, lies between layers of shale and sandstone. It is created by slow decomposition and compression of trees, ferns or mosses.

Metamorphic rock (basalt) is born of heat and pressure when igneous rocks are subjected to tremendous heat and pressure and become much harder. A metamorphic rock has undergone such changes. Many rocks are metamorphosed by heat and steam. Heat changes some materials, while steam makes others combine with materials from magma.

Volcanic stones are *orbicular* (having no single explanation of origin), containing concentric shells of different textures and mineralogy. Some are metamorphic rock that occurs at *convergent margins* (places where two tectonic plates collide). *Subduction* occurs, where the edge of one crustal plate is forced below the edge of another plate, producing high temperatures and pressurized environments deep within the Earth.

Mineral Content

The presence of certain minerals in metamorphic rocks can aid in their identification process. Garnet and kyanite, for example, occur in gneiss and schists, while crystals of pyrite grow on the cleavage surface of slate. Minerals such as brucite occur in marble.

Marble that has been formed consists mainly of calcite. Although pure marble is white, there are many variations. The impurity of mineral content may stain it to appear gray, yellowish, blue or pink; carbon may make it black. Marble is often used for tombstones, and was used for both the interior and exterior of the Supreme Court Building in Washington, D.C. Not usually recommended as a massage stone, its extreme capacity for retaining cold seems to be invasive when applied to delicate tissue.

Because it is so beautiful, jade is often classified as a gem, and it is associated with the five virtues: wisdom, justice, charity, modesty and courage. Although it is considered to have curative powers, jade is not recommended as a massage stone.

The igneous, sedimentary and metamorphic rock that makes up the Earth's crust is all formed from the same basic materials. The differences between them are due to the formation of each by a separate process. Rock formation is a slow process that has been occurring throughout time.

Rock formed directly from molten rock that cools quickly on or near the Earth's surface has a more *aphanitic* texture, so close that its separate grains are invisible to the naked eye. It can also have a distinctly rough lava texture, especially in some types of basalt.

The most common minerals in ingenuous and metamorphic rock can be identified by looking closely at their physical properties.

Igneous and sedimentary rocks cover about three-quarters of the Earth's surface and have long been associated with metal ores and extremes in texture, color and composition. Depending on their original region and mineralogy, these stones are well known for their heat- or cold-retention properties, making them a perfect choice for Stone Therapy.

* * *

Crystal Properties

"The basic block of minerals, oxygen and silicon"

Minerals containing sodium chloride and potassium are classified *electrolytes*. Two more, calcium magnesium and phosphorous, are major structural components of bone and teeth; phosphorus is also involved in the manufacturing of RNA and DNA for building new cells. Other electrolytes include iron, chromium, manganese and zinc.

Crystals contain unique properties, some of which are shared by all crystals, while others are specific to only certain ones. They are capable of generating a static charge through either heating or friction. An example is Stone Tapping with its resulting piezo electric effect as discussed in a later chapter, which produces energy (light). The expansion that follows compression releases electrons followed by re-absorption, creating energy.

These special qualities can be incorporated into strategies to attain wellness. Certain qualities function more on a physical-energy level while others function on a more vibrational level. Crystals' esoteric and physical properties are used worldwide.

* * *

Natural Permanent Magnets

Paleo magnetism is that acquired by a rock at the time of formation. The best-known natural permanent magnet is a ferrite, also known as magnetite or lodestone. Ferrites contain iron, oxygen and other elements.

Scientists who study the lava of ancient volcanoes have found that geomagnetic fields periodically reverse direction. When lava appears on the surface, it cools gradually, locking in the Earth's magnetism. When the lava has completely cooled, it forms a stone containing the magnetic energy of the Earth. However, it is the iron (ore) content of the volcanic stone that will establish its magnetic power and its durability as a heat-retaining agent in Stone Massage. Lava leaves a record of the geomagnetic field at the time the lava cooled, individualizing each stone.

Special Stones Used for Stone Massage

The powerful metathetic energies of these unique stones are well known to promote a harmonizing and balancing effect when used with massage, allowing a meditative state of quietude and calm to evolve. The application of hands in conjunction with stones intensifies these effects, increases universal energy, assists with the energy flow within and directs that vital energy to areas of blockage.

The initial imprint of magnetic energy during rock formation and specific mineral composition seem to be strong determining factors for stones selected for Stone Massage therapy. Another is the ability to maintain proper temperature. The ability or inability to retain heat consistently can be the difference between a phenomenal treatment and a possible injury from burning.

Correct mineralogy is also a significant determining factor in the energy directing and transference process. To achieve the maximum effect, all stones should be naturally smooth and unaltered. I personally do not use or recommend mechanically altered stones because I do not feel they are conducive to Stone Therapy. Research indicates that this process prevents the stones from accepting heat evenly and they do not heat properly. The process also seems to interfere with energy transference.

When the exteriors of stones have been altered through tumbling and polishing, they also become more difficult for the practitioner to manipulate. Polished stones can become very slippery, especially after lubricant is applied, which should always be used in conjunction with Stone Therapy.

Selecting and collecting stones from only certain regions because of their durability as a heat-retaining agent is important due to paleomagnetic properties. As discussed earlier, stones originating from volcanic eruptions cool extremely quickly, thus securing within them Earth's magnetism. Our Earth's geomagnetic field varies also, so the intensity of the geomagnetic field can increase in one region and be less severe in another. Certain stones high in magnetite, for example, are natural magnets because they are formed in a specific area.

For many years, I experimented with a wide variety of stones to find the suitable combination for therapy. I concluded that smooth basalt volcanic stone was most conducive to warm therapy. For cold therapy, sedimentary stone was best, its primary origin being the cool waters of the ocean, rivers and lakes.

Using stones formed by sedimentary and volcanic action is very effective, not only because of the warm stone's thermal conduction effect that brings about local and systemic changes in the body, but also because it can influence energy centers to balance the body and mind. These smooth, volcanic basalt stones easily convey warmth to the skin, greatly increasing circulation. Warm basalt stones profoundly relax the client at the deepest level almost immediately.

Great pressure and high temperatures deep within the Earth can alter existing rocks and create new ones. In the basalt, this sometimes involves only *smearing* (a deformation) or *breakage* of mineral formation, forcing the chemical components to reorganize into configurations that are stable under the new conditions. Other times, the change is so severe that mineral stability is affected, resulting in color variances ranging from light to dark gray or even black.

Basalt is a heavy, dark lava that is found the world over. It consists mainly of pyroxene and plagioclase feldspar, but the texture is so fine that these individual minerals are rarely visible. Basalt varies in color from dark gray with a greenish tinge to almost black.

Recently basalt has also been discovered on Mars. The *Sun-Sentinel* in South Florida reported on February 8, 2004, "Spirit Rover drills its first hole into rock on the planet Mars and could give scientist clues to Mar's geological past. The football-size rock is thought to be made of basalt, a volcanic material." That basalt has similar composition as our massage stones is very interesting, to say the least.

*   *   *

Chapter 6

ENERGY VORTEXES AND MANIFESTATIONS

My company chooses to import all our stones because we are committed to the industry and to this modality. Stones should be of a specific mineralogy originating from areas of high energy vortex (spectrum) and, of course, of unpolluted vastness. As conscious green-Earth advocates and environmentalists, we must be responsible enough not to deplete areas of their natural ecological environment for the sake of financial profit.

I find the finest quality stones conducive to Stone Therapy are harvested and imported from Argentina, Indonesia and Peru. These countries have regions of unusually high energy vortex where people feel a tremendous connection to the Earth. This energy is one of the primary reasons we import stones from the pyramids in Teotihuacán,

Mexico and Cairo, Egypt; Machu Pichu in Peru; Nepal; Greece; Thailand and others.

The Bermuda Triangle is famous for its high energy vortex and for the mysterious, unexplained disappearances of airplanes and ships.

Among the dramatic rock formations of the Cederberg mountain range in South Africa is the Maltese Cross, a 66-foot-high pillar. Consisting partly of Table Mountain sandstone and resistant to erosion, it forms the upper portion of the cross, which is richly colored by iron oxides.

Cuzco in Peru (The Capac Usnu) was among the greatest wonders of the ancient world. For the Inca, it was literally the sacred center of the universe. There is also compelling evidence that the Incas practiced herbal medicine and shamanistic healings at times in which they included semi-precious stones. Peru is recognized for its areas of high radiance spectrum.

There are several vortex sites in the United States. Sedona, Arizona has seven sites used by ancient tribes for rituals and ceremonies, as well as its magnificent red rock desert. Another such area is the Serpent's Mound in Adams County, Ohio where my family first settled.

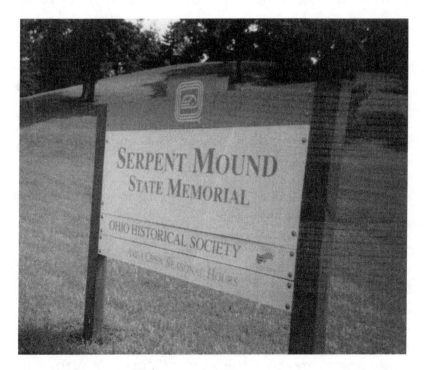

The Serpent Mound

Art that has been recovered from the Mississippi Valley dates back further than in any other region of the United States, the earliest works being massive earthworks. The Serpent Mound in Ohio is perhaps the best-known of these, and has the largest and finest effigy mound in the world.

Serpent Mound is situated in Adams County, a few miles from the village of Loudon on State Route 73. Stretched along the east bluff of Brush Creek, the mound is an embankment of earth nearly a quarter-mile long representing a gigantic serpent in the act of uncoiling. The body of the serpent extends in seven deep curves nearly to the tip of the elevated bluff on which it lies. An oval wall of earth separate from the mound forms the body and represents the serpent's open mouth.

While some people were hoping to discover evidence of a lost civilization such as Atlantis, others were studying the Serpent Mound in present-day Ohio. Serious researchers became certain that it was created by ancestors of the Native Americans who were occupying North America when the first Europeans arrived.

Archaeologists found that two small conical mounds and one large one south of the effigy contained burials and implements characteristic of the prehistoric Adena Indians. The Adena people probably built the mound sometime between 1000 B.C. and 700 A.D.

* * *

The Serpent is situated along the edge of a crater-like formation that may be evidence of a gigantic collision between the Earth and an asteroid or meteor. Geologic evidence in the form of disturbance patterns in underlying rock and carbon tests of charcoal found within the mound indicate it was created about the same time that Haley's Comet passed over the Earth.

The high ridge on which it lies is part of a ring graven where rocks were dropped after a gigantic explosion some 200 million years ago in what is now Ohio. The resulting ring, 3.5 to 4 miles in diameter, is called the Serpent Mound Crypto explosion structure.

Excavations of the Serpent Mound did show that the serpentine form had been carefully planned before the mound was built. Flat stones and lumps of clay were laid on the ground surface as a guide, and baskets of earth were piled over them.

Serpents have figured prominently in the religions of many world civilizations. To many ancient people, they represented eternity because the annual shedding of their skin seemed a renewal of life. In the myths and ceremonial practices of American Indians, serpents were sometimes considered beneficial and sometimes evil. The well-known Snake Dance of the Hopi Indians of Arizona is celebrated chiefly as a prayer for rain.

There can be no doubt that serpents symbolized some religious or mystical principle for the builders of Serpent Mound. The great size of the effigy mound indicates that the serpent was a very important factor in their belief system. The interpretation most frequently given to the mound is that it represents a gigantic serpent in the act of swallowing.

Some authorities who have drawn reconstructions of the mound believe the effigy represents a serpent striking while ejecting an egg, the oval earthwork. Other experts have thought that the oval symbolized the heart of the reptile or interpreted it as a conventionalization of the head and eye. However, more recently it is believed that the hinged jaw is open and that the oval earthwork is actually the mouth of the serpent about to clamp down.

Hill worship followed stone worship, and the first hills to be venerated were large stone formations. It became the custom to believe that the gods inhabited the mountains, so that high elevations of land were worshipped for this reason as well. As time passed, certain mountains were associated with certain gods so they became objects of worship and burial sites.

Long known by early settlers, Serpent Mound was first surveyed by Ephraim G. Squire and Edwin H. Davis in 1846. Then in 1886, Frederic W. Putnam of the Peabody Museum at Harvard University became interested in the site and succeeded in raising sufficient funds to purchase it and turn it over to the Peabody Museum. Under Dr. Putnam's direction, excavations and reconstructions of the Serpent and the three adjacent comical mounds were completed. In 1900, the entire area was deeded to the Ohio Historical Society, which now maintains the site.

The mysterious Serpent continues to encourage imaginative theories. In 1970, Erich von Däniken's book titled *Chariot of the Gods* suggested it was a signpost for aliens from outer space in the first book to introduce the theory that ancient Earth had been visited by aliens. Even today, people come to the site to watch the sunrise over the Serpent on the morning of the Summer Solstice, believing the Serpent marks a place on the planet that has special mystic vibrations. Coincidentally, geologists have determined that the site may actually have some kind of external atmospheric vibrations, and an extremely high energy vortex is located there.

As recently as September 14, 2003, the Ohio newspaper, *The Community Common* reported, "a strange design was found in a soybean field across from the entrance to Serpent Mound State Park on State Route 73 . . . remains under investigation . . . the design described as a crop circle." The site was inspected with a metal detector, revealing several metallic mineral levels, higher radiation levels inside the design, and higher electrical and magnetic fields inside than those outside the markings.

A final report of the findings of the investigation has not been released as of this writing. I can recall numerous UFO sightings in the late 1970s, in this vicinity, personally and by local authorities.

Serpent Mound State Memorial is open to the public year-round during daylight hours. Observation towers were constructed to permit visitors to look down on the mound and the surrounding countryside. Ohioans and others who visit Adams County have a unique opportunity to view this strange and wonderful relic of a culture that thrived in this state before recorded history began in North America.

This is the general area where I resided in the 1970s. I was particularly drawn to this area and spent many hours there in meditation. This was also the general area where I first heard about Chief, the old Indian healer from the Shawnee tribe. And we know there are no coincidences.

The initial stones I began to collect in my research came from this area. My family still lives in that region and when I visit, I always visit the Mound—it holds profound memories and enlightenment for me.

The Stones' Healing Touch

Let us examine different types of energy applications and their implications relative to Stone Therapy.

Through my use of non-invasive therapy, I have experienced the healing power of touch and its profound effect on us and on those we touch. Did you know that an infant deprived of touch will die?

Stone Massage has been a part of my holistic regime for many years. This unique therapy utilizes basalt (warm), sedimentary (cool) and semi-precious stones; crystals; aromatherapy and corresponding Chakra placement. Although it is a physical practice, it has a vital spiritual root.

I have had the privilege of incorporating a wide range of modalities into my practice and teachings. Over the years, however, I have found that the most powerful influence, both internally and externally, is Stone Therapy. The remedy of ancient stones comes from the Earth, a spiritually rewarding experience aligning us on the road to renewal.

When practitioners use specific stones in conjunction with massage, they seem to tap into various vibrational frequencies. This invisible energy within our physical form is similar to electromagnetic induction, allowing the body's response to be mirrored back on the recipient. This information serves as a guide for the practitioner as to the appropriate mode of treatment. In this way, the body determines the electromagnetic shift needed to restore balance. New fields of quantum physics describe the human factor in the equation--the underlying nature of energy in relation to our own physical world.

Everything is made of vibrational energy. Photon particles are messengers, processing both strong and weak forces on a sub-atomic gravitational level. An atom's outer shell has a negative charge — inside is the nucleus. The mass of an atom is concentrated in the central nucleus made up of positively charged protons and neutral neutrons. Presently, we will consider the wider implications and endless possibilities.

The human energy system is viewed with a predominant frequency of energy. Everything in our world – animal, plant, even stone – vibrates and oscillates to some degree. Energy systems are capable of absorbing energy if it is introduced in a mutual resonating frequency. The human body has its own inherent frequency. Its vibrational rate can be a reflection of the body's current health.

Specific stones provide a resonant energy transfer to the recipient of the treatment, initiating a healing response in the body in the form of various energetic and molecular aspects, which vary from person to person.

I find it is not always crucial to understand all the elements of how something works in order for it to be a valuable modality. The truth lies in the outcome. Clients again and again share their wonderful experiences, from deep relaxation to a greater sense of well-being to life-altering changes, as a direct result of Stone Therapy treatments. They rarely expect the powerful impact of energy rebalancing and its effects on their physical as well as ethereal body.

Healing is derived from within, leaving us physically energized and spiritually aligned yet keenly aware that we are organic beings in a constant state of change. As we begin our journey with this ancient way of healing, be patient and gentle with yourself and feel your reconnection with the Divine Universal Energy, our higher state of being.

You will notice as you proceed that things will naturally come together. You may also notice that you are learning to exist on a deeper level of self. To heed this modality's true spiritual meaning, you will introduce a more vivid experience of spirit to the exploration of your inner world. You will make choices that nurture you and me in balance with the flow of the Universe.

We live in an energy field generated by the Earth, which influences many components on our planet, both living and non-living. As we shall now see, the stones used for Stone Therapy and their potential healing abilities are quite unique.

* * *

Chi Energy Channels

Chi is the life force energy
surrounding all living and inanimate things.
It takes on many forms, including rain, wind, snow
and sunlight.
Chi can be likened to a giant spinning whirlpool.
Indeed, if you stop and take the time to look
at what nature has created,
from the pattern inside a tree
to the delicate lines of a seashell to human DNA,
you will see this pattern constantly repeated.
This is truly the force of life,
evident in the beliefs of a multitude of cultures
both primitive and contemporary.
The *spiral* was symbolic of a variety of things
and a passageway to another place of transition
between the physical and spiritual realms.
It signified life, breath.
The essential purpose behind Feng Shui is to keep
Chi flowing smoothly and purposefully in a balance
of Yin and Yang energies.

Yin and Yang

Yin and *Yang* are the governing energy within the universe, flowing as a distinct pattern from organ to organ as opposite but complimentary forces.

The characteristics of Yin are darkness, cold and passiveness (female negative), signified by the color black. Yang represents lightness, heat, activity and excessiveness (male positive), represented by the color white. The anterior (front) surface of the body is considered to be Yin (cold) while the posterior (rear) is Yang (warm).

This energy begins at conception and remains within us throughout our life. The Yin male energy, that which is supportive and strong, balances with all things. Yang is a receiver of light energy and openness to be of service. The relationship of nutritive *qi* to defensive *qi* is a fundamental expression of Yin and Yang.

Meridian Theory

A healthy body is one in which the energy (Chi) is balanced and free-flowing through fourteen invisible channels called *meridians*. All channels begin and end in the feet and hands. Chi manifests itself as five interrelated elements; humans are considered a combination of all five.

When vital energy becomes imbalanced, bodily disorders develop. Balance needs to be restored to allow the body to correct the problem. As the energy stagnates along the channels at *tsulo points*, pain or tenderness indicates the energy imbalance. Stone pressure applied to the appropriate point manipulates and releases the energy to bring about balance and restore health.

Each meridian supplies a muscle group and internal tissues. Of the fourteen meridians, twelve are major or *organic meridians* and two are known as *storage meridians*.

Six of the organic meridians are called Yin meridians, which transport a negative-charged electromagnetic energy throughout the body and supply the Yin organs: heart, liver, lungs, spleen, kidney and circulatory vessels.

The other six organic circuits are referred to as Yang meridians, which transport the positive-charged electromagnetic energy throughout the body to the Yang organs: stomach, large and small intestines, gall bladder, urinary bladder and adrenal glands.

The two remaining storage meridians flow through the central body, along with seven glandular centers or *Chakras* that align along these two channels as *transducers.* They are actuated by power from one system and supply power, usually in another form, to a second system. This flow is called the *creation cycle* or *sheng cycle.*

When these subtle channels are blocked or unbalanced, due to stress for example, illness can result. Rebalancing these internal energies promotes health and well-being.

When unblocking the meridians, the speed of conduction can be almost instantaneous, but not for the blood and lymphatic system, which respond on the *cutaneous* (external skin) or *visceral* (internal organ) *reflex* level. Stimulating the skin has an effect on internal organs and other parts of the body. When it is applied at congested or painful places, therefore, it corresponds to the simplest form of acupuncture in which only the *locus dolenti* and not the distant part is stimulated.

The changing rhythm in the balance of Yin and Yang ensures that there is never an excess of either of these polar opposites, for over-activity of Yang is adjusted at once and automatically by the yielding passivity of Yin.

The Stone Tuning System

Unlike acupuncture, Stone-Tonics is an energy-based, non-invasive treatment. Crystals, warm and cool stones are applied on acu-points and the stones tapped rhythmically to address the body's meridians and Chakra energy systems. Their resonances and vibrations connect with and support the body's natural frequencies. They can also act as sonic enzymes, mediate between varied energy realms within us, and help to ground and root energy in the body.

Every stone has a component of crystals, hundreds of different elements including silicon. When tapped, they transmit subtle electro-magnetic energies. Silicon is a very important component of both crystal and our bodies.

Piezo Electricity Effect

Applying pressure to quartz crystals generates electric current in a phenomenon called *piezo electricity* (from the Greek word *piezein that* means "to press"). This principle is demonstrated by a piezo acu-stimulator such as the Acu-Spark, a handheld electric probe that generates current through crystals under pressure, stimulating specific acu-points to relieve pain.

When tapping two stones or crystals together, we release a burst of an electro-magnetic sound wave that connects with and helps the body's natural frequencies flow freely. We are thus brought into alignment with the source of original harmony, promoting healing on a deep cellular level.

When the stones are tapped together, one end develops a positive electrical charge while the other develops a negative one. Conversely, if pulled apart the electric charge changes its direction or polarity. In this way, stones are energy transmitters – they create balance and harmony by moving energy from where it is excessive to where it is lacking.

Science has shown us that if a crystal is placed in an energy field, it collects that energy, changing and transmitting it in the process. Quartz and many other crystals amplify energy and then radiate it out.

Black crystals, however, react somewhat differently. They absorb but do not release the energy in quite the same way, providing protection from negative sources and repelling unwanted energies when attuned properly.

These semi-precious stones are mined around the world, each with a distinctive coloration pattern reflecting its unique Earth element composite, each with its own story of the great geological changes of our planet over the past million years.

Through indirect mechanical and thermal effect, the piezo electrical effect increases the rate of chemical reaction within cells to facilitate healing, adjust local pH balance to less alkaline and more acidic, and increase the permeability of skin cells.

When effecting change on a cellular level, the body needs sufficient time to adjust to the process. You can aid it by remaining calm and by drinking adequate water. Remember, when you feel thirst, it is a message that your tissues have already become dehydrated. Do not wait.

During an earthquake, pressure on crystalline rocks can create the piezo electric effect when these non-conducting crystals become physically strained and electrically polarized. Changes in geomagnetic field fluctuation (GMF) are related to shifts in the Earth's tectonic plates.

These changes occur especially if magnetic-rock changes are involved and are influenced by the tectonic plate shift.

Modern western research shows that biochemical structures like bone and muscle act as a piezo electrical crystal, converting sound waves to electrical signals and providing a mechanism by which valuable change might be induced. To use this technique, firmly place a warm stone on a specific body area. With a second stone, tap the stone that is resting, while maintaining constant pressure into the muscle and making certain you are on the trigger point.

This form of treatment is also very effective when combining warm and cold stones. When tapping the stones above the body for energy release, the temperature of the stones is of no consequence.

Chapter 7

ELECTROMAGNETISM

Acu-Points

In all imbalances, whether physical or mental, there are tender areas at certain points on the surface of the body. When balance is restored, the tenderness dissipates. The Chakras similarly correspond to acupuncture points, or *acu-points*.

The specific points used in judo are also acupuncture points, which can cause a person to faint if too strongly stimulated. Sometimes a medical system indigenous to one part of the world seems mystical to people in other parts of the world. In reality, these systems portray many of the laws of nature, despite their expression in a language or manner that some might view as unscientific.

Magnetic Effects on the Body

The Earth is a great natural magnet with north and south magnetic poles, a magnetic axis and a field force that extends into outer space. The magnetic field on the surface of the Earth, or *geomagnetic field,* has strength of about ½ *gauss.*

The Earth's inner structure creates the geomagnetic field. Scientists believe it comes from the circulation of molten rock in the Earth's outer core. The inner core consists mainly of solid iron, which is highly conductive. Whether from natural or manufactured magnets or from the magnetic force of the Earth itself, the Earth's magnetism has a profound and direct influence on our health and well-being.

Magnets have been used in many parts of the world for centuries to relieve pain and to enhance the body's natural healing powers, with dramatic results. In modern medicine, studies have shown magnets to be an effective therapy to improve the body functions that affect energy. Many believe that applying magnetic fields to a body area increases blood flow and oxygen exchange for that area.

Indigenous healers were tested in modern scientific laboratories to verify the Chi that they claimed to emit. Results showed that these healers produced strong *infrasonic* sound waves (below the range of the human ear) from their hands. Further testing proved substantial beneficial changes in the electroencephalogram (EEG) tests of their subjects.

To understand the critical role that magnetic energy has in relation to human health, we must begin with our body's true multidimensional spectrum. This includes not only biomagnetic energies generated by cellular activity within our body, but also subtle magnetic energies related to Chakra and meridian activity and the body's field of aura. If we add to this our planet's magnetic energy and vast electromagnetic pollution, we can begin to see the complexity of the issue. Varied energy fields can be powerful tools to effect change on many levels of the living system we call The Human Body.

There are theoretically about 5.5 million single-domain magnetic crystals in each gram of human brain tissue and 120 million magnetic crystals in each gram of the *pia* and *dura mater* that envelops the brain. These crystals in turn contain particles of *biogenic* magnetite formed by living organisms within body tissue.

* * *

Electromagnetism and Healing

Electromagnetism refers to both the magnetism produced by electricity and the branch of physics that studies it. It is based on the facts that (a) an electric current or a changing electric field produces a magnetic field and (b) a changing magnetic field produces an electric field.

Electromagnetism is one of the basic forces in the universe and can be observed in nature in the common occurrence of lightning.

We are surrounded and activated by an electromagnetic field that influences the body through the infinite process of *photon* exchange. In this colossal electromagnetic energy field, the head and the right side of the body represent the positive electrical pole, while the feet and the left side represent the negative pole. The spine – the central core of the body – represents neutral but carries within its cerebra-spinal fluid the most potent of all energy flows: the Kundalini.

In the human energy field, electromagnetism circuitry is ever-present. Electrical force is responsible for holding together all the atoms and molecules from which matter is composed, and is associated with many biological processes. Electrical signals travel along our nerves, carrying information to and from the brain. They tell the brain what the eyes see, what the ears hear and what the fingers feel.

When stress and chemical imbalance are present in any part of us, they alter the *ionic matrix* of our energy field, where an atom or group of atoms originates, and will likely result in an overly positive ionic charge. This is why some healings can occur naturally after spending time in natural surroundings such as at the seashore or in the mountains. The plentiful negative ions in those atmospheres help to normalize our circuitry. Nature surrounds us – collectively we are part of it.

Distinguishing ourselves from nature is like attempting to separate a wave from the ocean.

The powerful transformation energies of Stone Massage contribute to healing by imparting their natural antidote to ionic distortion and disorders. Since all ions are governed by polarity principles and possess either a positive or negative charge, specific stones when tapped can resonate and transmit energy.

The electromagnetic field of the body can be seen with the use of *Kirlian photography* mentioned earlier and named for its 1939 Soviet inventers. It is done very close to the body, directly over the skin, and can stretch 4 to 5 cm outward (up to two inches). In this field, the entire momentary condition is pictured but it can change in an instant.

The Chakras and Their Stones

For thousands of years,
stones have been used for healing.

The ancient art of crystal healing uses the gentle transformation properties of stones and semi-precious stones. Specific resonance of these transmits energy: this is the premise of the Stone Massage Chakra Balancing treatment. Specific mineral stones placed on specific points of the body are capable of dissolving stress, removing blockages, neutralizing negative energies, drawing energy away from over-stimulated areas and re-energizing a depleted one, thus inducing a feeling of well-being and balance.

By virtue of their beauty, these stones are much more than ornamental in function. In Asiatic religions, they symbolize the treasures of correct religious teachings. Jade, for example, in its countless varieties is a symbol to the Chinese of multiplicity and infinity.

The Seven Chakras

The Journey to Enlightenment

©2002 Sonia Alexander, Inc.

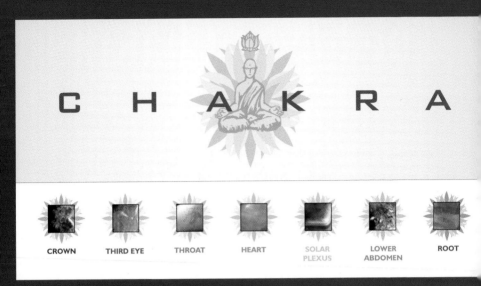

C H A K R A

| CROWN | THIRD EYE | THROAT | HEART | SOLAR PLEXUS | LOWER ABDOMEN | ROOT |

DIRECTING THE VITAL ENERGY FLOW WITH STONE TAPPING, CLEANSING, ACTIVATING, BALANCING AND ALIGNING EACH SPECIFIC CHAKRA SITE.

Vital health requires the free flow of life force between the seven major Chakras (energy centers)
Each of these spinning wheels exhibit a different quality of energy, governing
the process of that particular Chakra center.

EASTERN VIEW

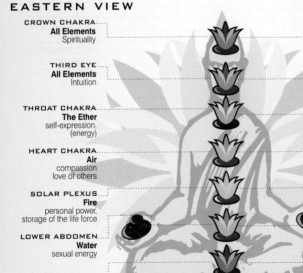

CROWN CHAKRA
All Elements
Spirituality

THIRD EYE
All Elements
Intuition

THROAT CHAKRA
The Ether
self-expression,
(energy)

HEART CHAKRA
Air
compassion
love of others

SOLAR PLEXUS
Fire
personal power,
storage of the life force

LOWER ABDOMEN
Water
sexual energy

ROOT CHAKRA
Earth
the lower limbs

WESTERN VIEW

BRAIN
Triggers relaxation
response

PITUITARY GLAND
May signal glands
to secrete fewer
stress hormones

THYROID GLAND
May signal glands
to secrete fewer
metabolic hormones

HEART
Strengthens circulatory
system, lowers
blood pressure

LUNGS
Improves deep
breathing

ADRENAL GLANDS
May deactivate
stress response by
suppressing adrenalin

KIDNEYS
Enhances drainage
of waste from lymphatic
system

REPRODUCTIVE ORGAN
May influence secretion
of sex hormones

Made in USA by Sonia Alexandra © 20

Throughout the world, crystals occurring gem-like in nature have symbolized perfect virtue. In Christian symbolic representation, for example, rock crystal was associated with the Virgin Mary because it is not a source of light itself, yet sparkles when a beam of God's light strikes it.

Reflective gems, especially crystals, were often used as aids to meditation and were believed to have healing properties. The ability of crystals to focus energy means they can be used for specific tasks. Crystals also have a more prosaic application: they can be found in every segment of society, storing and focusing energy. They cut, transmit, absorb and regulate. Quartz crystal powers our watches, controls our computers, emits radio waves – our world could not function without them.

Chakras, meaning *wheels* in Sanskrit, are energy points linking the physical body with electromagnetic energy. If blocked or overactive, Chakras create disharmony within us.

To balance the Chakras, the appropriate semi-precious stone is placed on each Chakra site. These stones can be placed on the front, back or both – the level of training and mode of treatment will determine the technique to be used by the practitioner.

There is one central underlying energy process in the physical body. This is difficult for us to comprehend. To eliminate confusion, let us simply accept that any given energy is what it is, regardless of what form or psychological impact it has at any given moment.

Another energy, the *Chi Body*, exists within the same space as the physical body just beyond the skin and is also known as the *aura*. It vibrates at a higher frequency than the physical body, the level at which Stone Chakra Bio-Resonance works. Simply holding a quartz crystal at least doubles the aura, an effect that can be captured by *Kirlian photography*.

Still another and subtler body energy of even higher frequency than the aura is the Emotional Body. It is believed to extend far beyond the physical body to the outer bounds, a higher consciousness. All emotional experiences are stored within the body.

The seven Chakra sites of the body are vortexes, like whirlpools through which energy transformation occurs. The use of specific mineral stones associated with each Chakra and the quality attributed to each of those stones aids in the stimulation and balancing of the Chakras. Traditional Chakra theory stems from the premise that *Kundalini energy* sits near the Root Chakra at the base of the spine. When the higher Chakras are also awakened and in balance, the Kundalini energy can rise unhindered to awaken your full potential and aid in attaining enlightenment, a complete spiritual unfolding.

Another method to open a Chakra is by rotating a quartz wand in a counterclockwise direction, while closing it is by rotation in the opposite direction. This method is a suggested way to begin. The energy rotation of one's Chakra is not always consistent between males and females. On an advanced level, the focus is on the Kundalini energy located at the base of the spine and the importance of intuitively feeling the energy direction and rotation of each Chakra prior to the actual release sequence.

* * *

Listed below are the seven Chakra locations and the semi-precious stone that I personally found to be most effective when working with each one. Also included is a brief history and description of each stone. In addition to the quality listed for each Chakra arrangement, the body organ in the area of each Chakra can also be addressed with stones exhibiting the colors associated with said Chakra.

1. Location: Root   Origin: India, Brazil, Mexico
   Gemstone: Bloodstone   Color: Green
   Description: Bloodstone, also called heliotrope, is a dark green, translucent chalcedony. The green color results from densely packed mossy crystal growths called dendrites. Speckled throughout the lovely green color are tiny spots of red and jasper that resemble drops of blood from which this stone gets its name. Bloodstone has been popular as a semi-precious gemstone for thousands of years, many legends are associated with it and it is a birthstone for March, realigning lower Chakra energies.

2. <u>Location</u>: Lower Abdomen <u>Origin</u>: Worldwide
   <u>Gemstone</u>: Jasper <u>Color</u>: Varied
   <u>Description</u>: Jasper ("Supreme Nurturer") is a forum of quartz (silicon dioxide) containing so much variance that light no longer passes through it. The impurities may cause jasper to display as either red, yellow, brown, green or grayish-blue. Bloodstone is a well-known form of jasper. A most unusual color occurred when deposits of red and yellow jasper were broken and fractured by ancient geologic upheavals and the pieces cemented back together by later deposits of lighter-colored chalcedony. This form of jasper is called brecciate (broken up) jasper and results in some very unusual and beautiful patterns.

3. <u>Location</u>: Solar Plexus <u>Origin</u>: South Africa
   <u>Gemstone</u>: Tiger's-eye <u>Color</u>: Varied
   <u>Description</u>: Tiger's-eye is quartz (silicon dioxide) with inclusions of other minerals, which produces its shimmering play of colors and iron, which causes brown and red colors. The natural

colors of tiger-eye are gold, red and blue. This stone brings clarity of intention.

4. Location: Heart   Origin: Brazil, Namibia
   Gemstone: Rose Quartz   Color: Pink
   Description: The beautiful color of this quartz is probably caused by tiny amounts of manganese. It is frequently used as a semi-precious gemstone and sometimes as a meditation stone, aiding in deep inner healing.

5. Location: Throat   Origin: Zimbabwe
   Gemstone: Turquosite   Color: Blue
   Description: Naturally milky white in color, this copper and phosphate mineral is dyed to give it the lovely blue color that resembles turquoise, a rarer stone often used by the Indians of the southwestern United States for jewelry and medicine pouches. The mineral name for this stone is howlite or magnetite. Good quality is rare. Turquosite is a problem-solving stone.

6. Location: Third Eye   Origin: Brazil

   Gemstone: Sodalite   Color: Blue

   Description: Sodalite is a complex sodium aluminum silicate with chlorine resembling lapis lazuli in color. As an igneous mineral, it is formed as molten rock cooled slowly deep in the Earth. Some specimens are fluorescent under ultraviolet light. This stone creates objectivity to intuitive processes.

7. Location: Crown   Origin: Brazil, Africa

   Gemstone: Amethyst   Color: Purple

   Description: This tumble-polished stone is a semi-precious variety of quartz (silicon dioxide). The purple color is probably due to traces of manganese. Amethyst occurs in hollow gas tubes in ancient lava flows. It is a very popular gemstone and is the birthstone of February. This stone cleanses the aura and protects it by drawing in divine energy.

Chapter 8

APPLICATIONS AND TREATMENTS

Examples of Semi-Precious Stones and their Purposes

<u>Pink Kunzite</u> is the perfect stone for healing the heart. It activates the heart Chakra, purifying and filling it with peace, and removes emotional debris left behind from past relationships.

<u>Rose Quartz</u> is the stone of unconditional love. Soft pink in color, it gently dissolves blockages to love.

<u>Black Tourmaline</u> deflects and repels negative energy, especially psychic attack, and protects against ill-wishers.

<u>Tiger's-eye</u> grounds, centers and brings awareness of one's needs.

Citrine stimulates openness and helps solve problems.

Aventurine releases anxiety, boasts tranquility and promotes leadership skills.

Jade, a symbol of purity, protects and brings harmony.

* * *

Cleansing the Semi-Precious Stones

Immerse the stones in the ocean – a handful of sea salt works as well. Rinse them in water and dry. You can also place the stones in sunlight or store them in a sea salt container overnight to re-energize.

Certain stones resonate with the energy of the sun such as red, orange and yellow, while others such as white, green, blue and violet respond to the gentler energy of the moon.

To see an example of this use: Begin by placing a rose quartz stone in the area of the Heart Chakra between the warm torso placement stones and tap with an attunement wand to aid in balancing the Heart Chakra. The crystalline structure of the wand can absorb and transmit subtle electromagnetic energy.

The ability of crystals to focus energy means that they can be used for specific tasks such as directing healing energy to points on the body.

* * *

Chapter 9

THE EFFECTS OF STONE THERAPY

As you incorporate semi-precious stones into your Stone Therapy, please use caution as in most instances, the client will experience an emotional release. As stated earlier, always refer to your level of training. Do not attempt these procedures without adequate understanding and education about them.

Also, please note, as one becomes more attuned to the stones, intuition can also guide you to the most beneficial mineral and to the best location for its placement. When one uses these methods with loving intent, there can be no adverse effect.

What makes Stone Therapy so effective?

The physical body is one with the mind and emotions; they cannot be separated. Disharmony, either physical or emotional, within a person's energy system is expressed as disease. As discussed earlier and seen in the energy activity within our bodies, our vast electromagnetic circuitry is always present. An example is *ubiguinones,* a group of *lipid-solubles* used by every cell in our bodies. Vital to good health and survival, they are critical transporters of electrons and especially of *mitochondria,* our cells' fundamental powerhouse-generating body energy.

The powerful transforming energies from the stones, when combined with massage therapy, impart natural antidotes to disorders and ionic distortion to harmonize, restore and rejuvenate the body at the deepest level.

The temperature of the stone is transferred to the body by means of conduction. The longer the application, the deeper the penetration via reflex conductions to muscle tissue and joints. Penetration may reach up to 1.5 inches into the superficial layer of muscle. Following exposure to heat, the surrounding tissue may contain an excess of blood due to increased blood flow caused by a derivative response known as *vasodilatation.*

As blood leaves congested areas, there is a localized increase of capillary blood pressure. Red and white blood cells multiply, and for every 34 degrees Fahrenheit rise in internal temperature, metabolism increases by 10 to 15 percent. This occurs through broad application of warm stones to the body, which in turn aids in the treatment of weakened conditions by stimulation and detoxification.

Effects of Warm Stones on the Body

- Increase in heart rate and respiration
- Vasodilatation of capillaries
- Flexibility by relaxing of connective tissue
- Increase in metabolism and elimination
- Increase in migration of leukocytes
- Defense against infection

* * *

Effects of Cold Stones on the Body

The effectiveness of these sedimentary stones is attributed to their limestone mineralogy, which seems to enhance their cold-retention properties. They are harvested primarily from Indonesia and Argentina and are used only for cold, not warm, Stone Therapy. Originally formed deep within ocean basins, these stones came from plant life and coral reefs.

Prior to application, pre-cool these stones in a freezer or refrigerator and place them in a container with ice. Remove and blot the stones when you are ready to use them. Remember to handle the cold stones by their edges so that your own hands do not absorb the coldness of the stone and the client receives the full benefits.

Introduce the stone to the body with gentle tracing movements. Indication for local application to a specific body part includes early treatment of sprains, contusions, soft tissue injuries and certain arthritic conditions such as acute bursitis. The effects prevent swelling and relieve pain (cold receptors override pain transmission).

Deeper circular motion with a cool stone produces hyper stimulation, or analgesia. This allows the muscle to assume its normal relaxed state; i.e., normal phases, slight burning, aching and numbness. It is generally recognized that the 'pain gate' can be shut by stimulating the nerves that carry the signal to enable pain relief through massage and other techniques. Indications are over trigger points.

Cool Marine Stones are excellent for decongestion of specific areas. On deep tissue, for example, either orbital or sinus, they help in a safe and holistic way to reduce arrhythmia and soothe the irritation that often accompanies specific procedures.

When frozen or iced, cool stones have a silky texture that facilitates gliding manipulations without the use of a lubricant. Due to their mineralogy, when frozen or iced they will sometimes take on a green hue.

These lighter and more porous stones are extremely effective in the use of cold applications, producing constrictive action in the tissues. Please be aware that the cold stones will sometimes leave a slight red mark. They are not created by the same internal response as the ones left by the warm stones. It is due solely to the fact that the client has laid on them for a time, leaving an "imprint" from the pressure. These marks will disappear immediately after the stones are removed from the area.

* * *

Effects of Alternating
Warm and Cold Stones

The reflex effect of warm and cool stones can be used either to send blood to an *ischemic* area with too little, or to remove blood from a *hyperemic* (engorged) area. Adequate local application of warm and cold stones to the skin surface not only affects the immediate skin area, but also other areas in the body via the nervous system. The skin surface carries the stimulus along a nerve fiber to the spinal cord. From there the stimulus can travel to a related organ or elsewhere in the body. Generally, the skin area over an organ is in reflex relationship to that organ.

Alternating the application of warm and cold stones very effectively increases microcirculation and oxygen intake within tissue. When used in this manner, the stones can also effect change on a cellular level. Alternating vasodilatation with warm stones and constriction with cold ones produces decongestion of an area. Warm and cold are opposite, yet complimentary, forces. The systemic effect of cold increases the general metabolism while the systemic effect of heat has a sedative effect.

* * *

Effects on Body Systems

Circulatory System: Provides lymph drainage and toxin removal. Promotes thermo-genesis and cell hydration.

Musculoskeletal System: Increases range of motion. Nourishes intervertebral ligaments. Helps mobilize connective tissue. Softens elastin, collagen and adhesive tissue.

Nervous System: Calms the nervous system. Provides balance throughout parasympathetic system. Nourishes nerve cells.

Vascular System: Increases the flow and rate of blood circulation. Causes veins to dilate or widen.

Visceral/Organ System: Provides relaxation, decongestion and detoxification.

Emotional, psychological and spiritual needs of the recipient are all also addressed and benefit through Stone Massage.

* * *

Chapter 10

STONE THERAPY
PROCEDURES AND TREATMENTS

Contraindications

Although Stone Therapy can bring great improvements to the lives of many, it is critical that the practitioner knows when and to whom *not* to administer this treatment, as follows:

- Any condition where general massage is contraindicated

- Any surgery where nerves have been cut, causing a loss of feeling in areas

- Any disease where there is nerve damage or neuropathy (an abnormal and usually degenerative state of the nervous system or nerves); diabetes; osteoporosis.

- Any skin conditions which may be aggravated by moisture or heat

- Pregnancy; heat is the variable of concern. In the hands of a highly skilled therapist, treatment can be altered to a safe application, but never in the first trimester.

- Use of prescription medications with possible side effects due to temperature challenges or emotional distress

- Heart disease; temperature changes challenge the circulatory system

- A condition of extreme excess weight or obesity, increasing challenges to the heart

- Varicose veins; avoid heat, but minimal cold is beneficial; use derivative procedures

- Autoimmune dysfunctions such as chronic fatigue syndrome or any condition where the immune system is already taxed; a doctor's prescription is recommended

- Cancer or the thin skin of the elderly; approach with caution, lighter pressure and temperature

- Young children need very little to stimulate their systems; reduce the treatment duration and the temperature

* * *

Diabetes: Signs, Causes, Complications

Patients exhibiting classic signs of Type II diabetes are overweight, hypertensive and inactive. The condition usually results from decreasing tissue insulin sensitivity and degeneration of pancreatic beta cells related to a high-carbohydrate diet and inactivity. The result is a chain of pathological processes involving mobilization and deposition of fat. The worst complication is *vascular destruction* because of atherosclerotic placing. As peripheral blood vessels become blocked, especially those that supply nerves, characteristic changes occur in the feet and ankles.

Any disease that impairs sensation of joint receptors predisposes the joints to micro trauma and joint derangement. Diabetic arthropathy (joint disease) affects the feet and ankles predominantly, causing a tingling or burning in the feet, although true sensation actually decreases. Thus, Stone Therapy is strongly contraindicated.

Diabetes: Contraindicated for Stone Therapy

Type II or non-insulin-dependent diabetes mellitus (NIDDM) affects millions of people and the condition usually develops after age forty, and many patients who present for treatment of musculoskeletal or neurological conditions may actually be experiencing reactions to uncontrolled blood glucose levels. Unfortunately, as many as half of those with this potentially debilitating condition are unaware of it. Being familiar with the disease process will give the practitioner greater understanding of Stone Therapy contraindications.

* * *

Guidelines for
Stone Therapy Treatment

- Use only a heating unit designed specifically for Stone Therapy to maintain water temperature between 120-140° Fahrenheit (47-50° Celsius). Do not use an electric skillet, Crock-pot or hot towel caddy to warm the stones. Due to their chemical composition, <u>never</u> heat stones in a microwave.

- Fill the heating unit with water so that the stones are fully submerged. The recommended method used to warm the stones should always be water; no heating pads, please.

- Optional: You may add a very thin piece of cheesecloth to the bottom of the unit to reduce the noise level and to protect the bottom of the unit from scratches.

- Do not lift the stones out of the unit with bare hands. Especially if the stones' temperature is above that recommended, use insulated gloves or a wooden spoon.

- Never apply stones to anyone at higher than recommended temperatures.

- Read instructions thoroughly before applying stones to anyone.

- Always use the thermometer to determine the temperature of stones.

- Avoid bony surfaces to avoid unnecessary bruising.

- Wipe excess water from stones and your hands before application to a client.

- Always inquire of your client whether the temperature of the stone is comfortable.

- During treatment, adjust the temperature as needed.

- All contraindications for massage apply to Stone Massage.

- All draping procedures for massage apply to Stone Massage.

- Clean stones between sessions and at the end of the day (See procedure later in this chapter).

Please remember that Stone Therapy is an advanced modality involving application of extreme temperatures directly to skin. It should only be performed by certified professional therapists, or body workers, who also have a congruous understanding of both hot and cold therapy (hydrotherapy) and its effects on the body.

This book is not intended as a substitute for medical advice and treatment. The reader should regularly consult a physician in matters related to his or her health, particularly with respect to any symptom or ailment that may require diagnosis or medical attention.

Every effort has been made to insure the information given in this book is accurate. Due to differences in skills, tools and conditions, however, Sonia Alexandra Inc. disclaims liability for the actions of persons or organizations using this modality and for any injury or occurrence, whether physical or mental, to readers' clients or to themselves.

* * *

Preparations for Treatment

Materials required:

1. A heating unit designed for Stone Therapy (see above Guidelines)

2. Approximately forty (40) basalt stones of varying sizes; seven (7) Chakra stones and one (1) attunement wand

3. Two (2) sheets

4. One (1) bolster

5. Three (3) hand towels

6. Stone massage oil (see Lubricant below)

7. Massage table

Lubricant: The use of a lubricant suitable to Stone Therapy is of extreme importance. A carrier oil such as sesame, grape seed or almond oil is the perfect medium. Lotions, however, are not highly recommended since they tend to cool the stones too quickly and are not conducive to the smooth, gliding strokes that are required for this procedure.

I recommend a good quality stone massage oil infused with aromatherapy. My own favorite blend is a carrier oil of pure virgin sesame combined with a special mixture of essential oils of myrrh, jasmine and lemon grass. When the warm stone blends with this unique formula, the aroma released is pure bliss. Everyone loves it – I mean, *loves* it.

Aromatherapy: For centuries, a body of traditional knowledge has existed about the healing properties of fragrant essential oils. Qualities can be combined to increase the benefits of any technique. These oils from herbs, flowers, fruits, spices, resins and leaves are not only soothing and healing, but also beneficial to the skin, stimulating and moisturizing. The oils also stimulate receptors in the brain's limbic system that positively affect our emotional state.

* * *

Stone Massage Treatment:
Level I

The actual techniques described here are a culmination of many years of massage and stone work. Presented as a simple and efficient method, they are easily adapted and incorporated into any existing non-invasive practice by a body worker. Here you will find smooth integration and easy-to-follow guidelines.

This treatment can begin with the client in either the *prone* (face down) or *supine* (face up) position, which shall be determined by the therapist. Sequences are given for the prone position, but the order can be reversed to adapt to the supine position.

#1. Take a deep breath, set your intentions and let us begin.

Instruct your client to lie on the table in the prone position and place a medium hand towel over the *sacrum* (lower back).

Retrieve a stone from the heating unit that will be placed on the sacrum and place it on the towel, wrapping it to prevent heat from escaping.

Undrape the client's hands and feet.

Retrieve four (4) medium stones from the unit.

Gently place one stone in each palm of the client's hands and one stone on the bottom of each foot, re-draping as you go.

#2. Stand on the left side of the table.

Place your right hand over the sacral (lower back) stone and your left hand between the shoulder blades.

Begin gently rocking the client with your right hand while keeping the left hand stationary.

Continue for 1-2 minutes or until you feel as though you have connected with the client.

#3. Walk to the client's head and undrape the back, being careful not to move the sacral stone.

Apply stone massage oil to the client's back for approximately five (5) minutes using effleurage (long, smooth) strokes to lubricate.

Stop and retrieve two (2) medium stones, centering them in your palms.

Ask your client to take in a deep breath. As the client exhales, apply the stones using similar strokes up and down the back.

Circle the inside of the *scapula* (shoulder blade) several times.

Retrieve two (2) more medium stones.

Glide the stones between the shoulder blades and down the rib cage.

On the return strokes, insert your fingers between the ribs, ensuring that your pressure is in your fingers and not on the stone.

Repeat the fore-mentioned strokes a few times, retrieving two (2) more medium hand stones to complete the movements if judged necessary.

#4.   Cover the client's back with the sheet.

Walk to either side of the client and undrape the nearest leg.

Remove the stones from the hand and foot on that side.

Spread oil over the entire leg, in the same manner as for the back, for approximately two (2) minutes.

Retrieve two (2) small stones.

Apply one stone to each side of the Achilles tendon. Your thumbs should be centered on the leg.

Using small circular motions, glide the stones up the leg stopping just below the knee. Repeat this movement.

Next, using the flat portion of only one stone, glide the stone slowly and with firm pressure up the entire length of the leg.

Retrieve two (2) medium stones.

Lubricate the area, position the stones in the center of each palm and begin above the knee. Again, your thumbs should be centered on the hamstring (upper leg) group.

Using circular motions, glide the stones up toward the hip area.

Retrieve two (2) more stones and using effleurage strokes, work the hamstring group until these stones are cool.

#5.   Repeat Step #4 on the opposite leg.

Remember to remove the stone that you placed in the client's hand and on the client's foot, always placing used stones in a separate container for cleaning at the completion of each treatment.

#6.   Remove the sacral (lower back) stone from your client's lower back and set aside.

Re-check the temperature of the stones inside the heating unit using a thermometer and adjust as needed.

#7.   Turn your client over to the supine position (face up) and ask him or her to sit straight up, assisting if necessary.

Place a hand towel on the table beginning from the lumbar (lower back) area.

Retrieve six to eight (6 to 8) medium back stones from the heating unit. Depending on the size of your client, you may need to use more or fewer stones.

Arrange them side by side on the table beginning at the sacrum so they will align along the erector spinae muscles (along both sides of the spine) when the client is lying flat.

Cover the stones with a hand towel and assist the client to lay back flat on the table.

Ask the client if he/she is comfortable and adjust the stones as necessary.

<u>Be sure that the stones are not directly on the spinous processes. Never place the stones directly on the spine.</u>

#8. Place a hand towel over the torso of the client and retrieve all five (5) of the warm stones from the heating unit.

Place these stones along the center of the torso, from just below the navel to the center of the sternum (chest area).

Undrape the feet.

Place the small, cozy toe stones between each toe and recover the feet.

Place the third eye stone in the center of the forehead and the crown stone touching the base of the skull.

#9.   Go to either side of the client and begin with the nearest arm.

Spread oil over the forearm and massage using effleurage and petrissage strokes.

Retrieve two (2) small stones from the heating unit.

Place and hold one stone against the posterior side of the wrist at the wrist joint.

Using the other stone placed in the center of your palm, massage the inside of the forearm using effleurage strokes.

Turn the stone on its side and glide the stone up the muscle of the forearm from the wrist to the elbow.

Lubricate and repeat these movements on the other side of the forearm.

Rotate the client's arm to the head of the table and let it rest there for a brief moment.

Retrieve two (2) small palm stones from the heating unit.

Using the same placement of the stones as you did for the wrist, massage the bicep muscle (front of the upper arm) with a one-handed petrissage stroke.

Repeat the same movements for the tricep muscle (back of the upper arm).

#10. Repeat these movements on the opposite arm.

#11. Remove the stone from the forehead and lubricate the area.

Cradle the neck in your hands for about two to three (2-3) minutes.

Meanwhile, curl your fingers under the occipital (groove at bottom of skull) and apply gentle traction to the neck, releasing your pressure every fifteen (15) seconds or so.

Retrieve two (2) small stones from the heating unit.

Holding the stones on your fingertips, insert your hands under the neck.

Slowly bring the stones up the neck to the occipital area and gently massage this entire area. Caution is advised near any endangerment site, major blood vessels or nerve plexus.

Repeat this movement several times until the stones are cool.

Rotate the client's head to one side and begin to massage the exposed area using your thumb in small circular motions.

Use firm, even petrissage strokes on the upper shoulder area.

Retrieve two (2) more small stones from the heating unit.

Place one stone under the shoulder of one side of the client.

Now rotate the neck in the opposite direction of the shoulder under which you placed the stone.

With the other stone, gently massage the entire scapula (shoulder blade) area using gentle effleurage strokes.

Massage both the anterior and posterior sides.

Retrieve the stone from under the shoulder of the now-exposed side of the neck.

Repeat the above movements.

#12. Go to one side of the client and undrape the nearest leg.

Remove the toe stones from the foot.

Lubricate the entire leg using both effleurage and petrissage strokes.

Retrieve two (2) medium stones from the heating unit. Again, your thumbs should be centered along the center of the thigh.

Begin with small circular movement up the leg until you reach the greater trochanter (upper thigh).

Repeat until the stones are cool.

Next, using two (2) more medium palm stones, place the stones in the same positions as you just did.

Using firm, long, full strokes, glide the stones up the thigh until you reach the hip area.

Rotate the stones in your hands every four to six (4-6) strokes.

#13. Retrieve two (2) small stones.

Lubricate, place and hold the stones just above the medial and lateral maleolus (ankle) of the tibia and fibula bone. Again, your thumbs should be centered along the tibia bone (shin).

Using small circular motions, glide the stones up the leg until you reach the area just below the knee.

Repeat these movements several times.

#14. Repeat #11 and #12 on the opposite leg from which you are working.

#15. Move to the client's feet and gently massage each foot gently with one (1) small stone.

Place one (1) stone under the sheet and one (1) over it.

Massage the bottoms of the feet one at a time using small, circular strokes.

Retrieve the other stone and repeat on the opposite foot.

Place and hold a stone on the bottom of each foot for approximately one (1) minute.

Now retrieve two (2) medium stones and begin gentle (tragger) rocking movements with a warm stone in each hand, a slow circling over the entire circumference of the body.

Softly instruct your client to rest a few moments before getting up; he or she has just experienced a deeply relaxing process of release and re-balancing. A catalyst for change.

The Chakra Balancing Procedure

This treatment can either be combined with a Stone Therapy Treatment or offered as a separate treatment.

As discussed in detail in earlier chapters, ancient scriptures concerning medicine tell us that the human body has developed and is controlled by hundreds of electromagnetic fields, or energy centers. The seven primary centers, or Chakras, are linked to the body's two primary systems, the central nervous system and the endocrine system.

Each Chakra is said to align with a specific major nerve plexus and endocrine gland. Each of these vortexes (spinning wheels) represents a different variance of energy associated with each particular Chakra.

The Chakras serve as vital sensory feedback energy fields that govern physical and emotional expression as well as spiritual development.

Each Chakra uniquely represents a separate body of wisdom with different attributes, needs and purposes. When in perfect harmony, it is reflected by the peace, balance and harmony it brings to every area of life.

As a practitioner, while reading and studying this book, always refer to your level of training. You will become increasingly familiar each time you use these techniques, including energy transference. You will also develop a thorough understanding of each Chakra and its location, associated emotion, rotation, suggested stone and fragrance (essential oils).

Incorporating the healing properties of essential oils can increase the benefits of any Chakra balancing technique by soothing, balancing, healing and helping to create a stronger alignment between the physical and spiritual body. Scents also seem to stimulate receptors in the brain's limbic system, which affects the emotional state. I found this to be very beneficial during the many years of my own practice. This should not, however, prevent a practitioner from following another path. Individual needs differ, offering us the opportunity to personalize this treatment.

The goal of chakra balancing is, through deepest relaxation and energy transference, to aid in restoring, balancing and reconnecting a person to his or her innermost state of being, leaving him or her physically and spiritually aligned.

To repeat previous cautions:

- Explain to your client that this therapy is advanced and will likely result in some form of emotional release.

- Do not attempt this procedure unless you are properly trained and prepared.

Always begin this procedure by clearly setting your intentions.

You will need the seven (7) semi-precious stones (crystals) specifically related to each Chakra and one (1) attunement wand. The crystalline structure of the wand gives it the ability to absorb, focus and transmit subtle electro-magnetic energy, especially when used in conjunction with stone tapping.

Begin this procedure with the placement of the warm basalt stones sequence first, and then retrieve the seven crystals associated with the Chakras, gently placing them between the warm basalt stones on each corresponding Chakra site.

Then, holding the attunement wand in your hand, begin rhythmically tapping each stone in the appropriate opening spin direction. Always begin at the Root Chakra and slowly move up to each of the other Chakra sites.

After completing this sequence, return to the Root Chakra and place the appropriate semi-precious stone on top of the warm basalt stone.

Gently and intuitively, tap the stones with the wand rhythmically for approximately one minute. Again, consecutively move upward to each Chakra site slowly, tapping each area in the same rhythmic manner.

After completing the crown tapping at the seventh and final Chakra, remain still for a few moments and visualize the intent again.

Now gently move to the opposite end of the body and begin the re-closing process of each Chakra. Again, always begin at the Root Chakra and move up to each consecutive Chakra.

Rotating the attunement wand in the opposite direction, slowly spinning your way up to the crown Chakra in the gentle process of re-closing each Chakra.

Retrieve two (2) warm basalt stones from the heating unit and gently begin the stone bio-resonance.

Tap these two stones together rhythmically until you sense intuitively that the balancing procedure is complete, leaving the client spiritually aligned to the degree that he or she has allowed.

This concludes this segment of the Chakra balancing. Allow your client adequate time to process the treatment results with a transitional rest of at least 10 minutes after you have completed the procedure.

It must be noted that with this particular stone Chakra procedure, clients will frequently experience emotional releases, sometimes even 5 to 10 minutes after the procedure. Be prepared to follow normal guidelines and protocol: Do not enter the client's space unless so indicated, remain calmly reassuring and wait for a signal from them.

As body workers, we recognize that the body frequently represses traumas, which can be stored in areas of the body to the point of affecting our ability to feel. The Stone Chakra Treatment can be a catalyst in the release of blocked emotions.

*　*　*

Cleansing and Charging the Stones

Because the crystalline structure of stones and crystals can transmit or retain energy, it is important to clean and neutralize them after each treatment and at the end of a day of use.

Between sessions, take your container of used stones to a sink after completion of the treatment and sanitize the stones with anti-bacterial soap. Then replace them in the heating unit and reset to the recommended temperature. You may also sprinkle a tiny amount of sea salt into the final rinse water to clear the energy.

At the end of the day, turn off the heating unit. Remove the stones from the unit and place them in hot water with anti-bacterial soap or sea salt. Wash and rinse each stone individually and place them on a towel to dry. Empty the heating bin, spray it with alcohol and wipe it dry. Return the bin to the heating unit and replace the stones in the bin. Do not turn the unit back on until you are ready to use the stones for your next treatment.

Recharge the stones after cleansing, using one of the following methods:

1. You may immerse the stones in the ocean or use a handful of sea salt* mixed with water. Rinse them in this water and place them in sunlight or moonlight or store them in a container of sea salt overnight to reenergize them.

2. Place stones or crystals in a glass or clay bowl containing enough organic raw brown rice to cover them for 24-48 hours. The rice will absorb unwanted energy, leaving the stones balanced.

3. Burn sage or cedar while holding the stones over the resulting plumes of smoke. This is a purifying method used by Africans and Native Americans.

* Sea Salt is a crystalline compound (sodium chloride), a mineral and a constituent of ocean water. It can be used as a neutralizer, preservative or re-energizer. French Atlantic sea salt is considered by many to be the best, harvested by hand from the pollution-free Isle of Noimoutier off the coast of France. This salt is unrefined and not treated with heat as many other sea salts may be.

* * *

Final Words

Due to the current strong interest in Stone Therapy on a worldwide level, I have made an effort to present this book as clearly and simply as possible to make the information accessible to all who are interested, whether professional or layperson.

We have examined here together the ancient knowledge of a therapy that has been passed on from hand to hand, creating a fusion of past to present. We have created a modern-day Stone Therapy by exploring and implementing new techniques in the elimination of stress and pain, the healing of emotional and physical wounds, and countless other possibilities both visible and invisible.

Let us note once again what makes Stone Therapy so effective. We must understand that our physical body is inseparable from our mind and our emotions. Disease can be regarded, therefore, as an expression of some kind of disharmony, whether physical or emotional, occurring within a person's energy system.

As the body's vast electromagnetic circuitry is ever-present and magnetism impacts us profoundly on a daily basis, we are surrounded and activated by numerous fields that influence the body through infinite photon exchange processes. When stress or chemical imbalance is present in any part of us, it not only presents itself as a key factor in physiological imbalances in the body's entire eco-system, but it can alter the ionic matrix of the body's energy fields.

Touch research continues to support the efficacy of massage and healing touch with a wide range of clinical applications, including facilitation of growth and development, enhancement of immune function, and relief of stress, pain and depression.

The relationship between the body, its connective tissue and acupuncture meridians, which are the key to Traditional Chinese Medicine (TCM) concepts such as blockage of qi (energy) and restoration of energy flow.

In Stone Therapy, I believe that the impact of the treatment is partially dependent on the stone's mineral properties and response due to the electromagnetic wave transference. When tapping the stones, a medium is created by which both giver and recipient adopt a phase between each wave, thereby doubling the wave, reversing the phase, and changing the wave's amplitude to zero.

This may seem like an audacious proposal on my part. The other energy may come from gravitation—yes, gravitation—especially due to these stones' high density. The resulting effect is of the converting force as a stable and balancing influence.

These powerful transformational energies when incorporated with human touch impart their natural antidote to ionic distortion and disorders, leaving us restored, rejuvenated and balanced at our deepest level. In harmony.

I am stimulated to continue my vision and research, designed to encourage people from all nations to embrace their differences and similarities.

As this new modality continues to gain momentum, undoubtedly you will hear different points of view expressed to you from other sources. Hopefully, having absorbed the knowledge herein, from now on you will now feel confident enough to discern facts from mere speculation. While utilizing your unlimited choices, I hope you will reference back to the material presented in this book and consider it your base, your Stone Therapy foundation.

When we understand

that life is really about our spiritual
unfolding

that we have within our hands a huge world
of discovery

that there are many avenues that we can
take

that we can draw on the full stretch of our
capacity . . .

When we fully comprehend Stone Therapy's
impact as a powerful influence, affecting positive
change in such a wide spectrum of ways . . .

Then we can truly acknowledge that the
possibilities are endless.

I invite you to take this journey with me, one
stone at a time. Together, we can change the world.

Thank you for allowing me this opportunity
to share my Stone Journey with you.

Bibliography

ROCKS, MINERALS AND FOSSILS OF THE
    WORLD
by Chris Pellant
Little, Brown & Company Publishing, 1990
ASIN: 0316697966

THE ILLUSTRATED GUIDE TO CRYSTALS
By Judy Hall
Sterling Publishing, 2000
ISBN: 0806936274

GRAY'S ANATOMY
By Henry Gray
Courage Books Publishing, 1974
ISBN # 006273142-4

HARPER COLLINS ILLUSTRATED MEDICAL
DICTIONARY
Time-Life Publishing, 1993
ICBN #006273142-4

RELAXATION & STRESS REDUCTION
   WORKBOOK
By Matthew McKay et al
New Harbinger Publishing, 1998
ASIN: 1879237822

MASSAGE FOR PAIN RELIEF:
   A STEP-BY-STEP GUIDE
By Peijian Shen
Gaia Books, 1996
ASIN: 1856750523

YELLOW EMPEROR'S CLASSIC
By Ilza Veith
Press Edition, 1949

SYMBOLISM 2 WOMEN
By Barbara Walker
ISBN # 0-6250992-5

Glossary

acu-point any of the points where a needle is placed in the practice of acupuncture

alkaline containing large amounts of potassium or sodium carbonate

anterior toward or near the front of the body

aphanitic a dark rock of such close texture that its separate grains are invisible to the naked eye

atherosclerosis an arteriosclerosis characterized by fatty deposits in the arteries

aura an energy field or distinctive atmosphere said to emanate from a body and be visible to certain individuals with spiritual powers

basalt a dark, dense to fine-grained igneous volcanic stone made of pyroxene and labradorite

biogenic formed by living organisms

bio-resonance energy balancing techniques using sound waves, energy release and transfer

breakage alteration of mineral formation by pressure and high temperatures underground

capillary one of the smallest blood vessels connecting the larger arteries with venules (minute veins), forming an intricate network throughout the body for the interchange of substances such as oxygen and carbon dioxide between blood and tissue cells

carrier oil catalyst for transfer of one compound to another

causal body higher energy field or spiritual level

Chakra any of seven energy centers in humans

condyle rounded projection at the end of a bone resembling a knuckle

convergent tending to move toward one point or to approach each other

creation or sheng cycle power from one system and supply power, usually in another form, to a second system

cutaneous referring to the skin

derivative the instantaneous rate of change of one quantity of function with respect to another; or a substance made from another substance

dura mater tough fibrous membrane that envelops the brain and spinal cord outside the arachnoid and **pia mater**

effleurage long, gliding massage strokes

effigy mound representation or image of a person sculpted as a monument

electron an elementary particle of matter having a negative charge

electromagnetism a fundamental physical force that causes interaction between charged particles

enzyme any of various proteins originating from living cells and capable of producing certain chemical changes in organic substances

endangerment site any of certain body areas that warrant special precaution because of underlying exposed nerves, arteries or organs

erythema abnormal redness of the skin due to capillary congestion

esoteric understood by or meant for only a select group who have specific knowledge

fibula the outer and usually smaller of two bones of the lower leg, from knee to ankle

gauss centimeter-gram unit of a magnetic field

geomagnetic relating to the magnetic field of a material body; terrestrial magnetism; as in *geomagnetic field fluctuation* (GMF)

hyperemic engorged with blood

hydrostatic relating to fluids at rest or to the pressures they exert or transmit

hydrotherapy therapeutic use of water as in a whirlpool or bath

hypoxia deficiency of oxygen reaching body tissue

igneous formed by solidification from a molten state through volcanic activity

indigenous originating or living or occurring naturally in a particular environment

infrasonic a frequency below the audible range of the human ear

ionic matrix the point from which an atom or group of atoms originates

ischemia localized tissue anemia due to obstruction of the flow of arterial blood

Kirlian photography application of a high-frequency electric field to an object, radiating a characteristic pattern of luminescence that is recorded on film

Kundalini the life force lying at the base of the spine until aroused and sent to the crown

limbric system the group of brain components concerned especially with emotion

locus dolenti near an acupuncture point or congested area

leukocyte white blood cell

lipid-solubles any of various substances that are soluble in nonpolar organic solvents, and that, with proteins and carbohydrates, constitute the principal structures of living cells

medial pertaining to the middle

magnetic flux lines of force used to induce magnetism in a substance

meridian invisible channel through which Chi energy flows

Mesoamerica areas in southern North American (Mexico, Honduras, Nicaraqua) where advanced pre-Columbian civilization flourished

metabolism chemical processes in a living organism to provide energy for vital processes

metamorphic related to a change in a rock by pressure, heat, and water that results in a more compact and more highly crystalline condition

metasthetic somatism a series of metamorphic processes causing change in minerals and stones

mitochondria a part of cells that produces energy, rich in fats, proteins, and enzymes

moxibustion the burning of small cones of dried leaves (moxa) or other substances on the skin, generally at points used in *acupuncture*, to treat diseases or to produce analgesia

nerve plexus a network of nerves

neuropathy disease or abnormality of the nervous system

oncology branch of medicine that deals with tumors, including study of their development, diagnosis, treatment, and prevention

orbicular having no single explanation of origin

organic having properties of living organisms

oscillate to swing back and forth with a steady, uninterrupted rhythm; to vary between alternate extremes, usually within a definable period of time

oxidize to increase a positive charge by removing electrons

paleo magnetism the magnetization acquired by a rock at the time of formation

photon the quantum of electromagnetic energy having zero mass, no electric charge and an indefinite lifetime

pia mater meningeal envelope firmly adhered to the surface of the brain and spinal cord; see **dura mater**.

protist one-celled organisms, including protozoans, slime molds and certain algae, of Protoctista, a new taxonomic classification.

Piezzo electricity electric polarity produced in certain non-conductive crystals when subjected to pressure, strain, tapping or temperature elevation

quantum smallest amount of a physical quantity that can exist independently, especially a discrete quantity of electromagnetic radiation.

quartz very hard mineral of silica found in many rocks worldwide, including sandstone and granite; varieties include agate, flint, opal and rock crystal

qi *or ch'i* In Chinese philosophy, the ethereal substance of which everything is composed

resonate to correspond harmoniously

sacrum five fused vertebrae forming the posterior (rear) wall of the pelvis

scapula either of two triangular bones forming the back part of the shoulder; shoulder blade

sedimentary of organic or chemical origin, rock mostly formed in layers, often containing fossils, over million of years

silicate one of insoluble and complex metal salts combining silicon and oxygen

silicon a nonmetallic element occurring in the earth's crust in silica and silicates and used in glass, semi-conducting devices, concrete, brick, refractories, pottery and silicones; atomic number 14; atomic weight 28.086; melting point 1,410°C; boiling point 2,355°C; specific gravity 2.33

smearing deformation of rocks caused by pressure and high temperatures underground

stone tonics a stone tuning system using minerals to produce vibrational frequencies

subduction the process by which the earth's crustal plate results in one plate being drawn down or overridden by another

temazcal manmade clay or stone hut used for rituals

tibia the inner and larger of two bones of the lower human leg, from knee to ankle

tsulo point area of the body where stagnated energy collects along channels, causing pain and tenderness

transducers device actuated by power from one system and supplying power usually in another form to a second system

trigger point area of the body that is experiencing hyper-irritability, painful to the touch and de-activated by direct pressure and stretching

ubiquinones a group of **lipid-solubles** used by every cell in the body and vital to good health

vascular pertaining to vessels that carry fluids such as blood, lymph or sap through the body of an animal or plant

vasodilatation the relaxing or widening of blood vessels, which increases blood flow

visceral confined spaces that contain organs

vortex place that draws into its center all that surrounds it

Yellow Emperor ancient text of Chinese medicine

* * *

About the Author: Sonia Alexandra

As a leading developer of and authority on the world-renowned Stone Therapy concept, Sonia Alexandra is a visionary who excels in blending an array of cutting-edge concepts, products and technologies. Her holistic concept of mind and body utilizes a unified vision of physical and spiritual elements to enhance health, harmony and beauty.

Sonia is one of the pioneers and authorities in the exploding health and beauty industry with over thirty years' experience that began in 1972 as a licensed massage therapist. She continued her studies and went on to become licensed in esthetics, cosmetology and related fields. Her first dream was eventually realized when she owned and operated the first holistic day spa in the country, located in Massillon, Ohio. The year was 1979, and Sonia added many more facilities in the following years.

Sonia's unique path has given her the forum to explore her innovative approach to health, wellness and beauty. It also maintains her inherent appreciation for the difference between a fashionable trend and the holistic mind-body approach to beauty and health.

Sonia Alexandra is the President of Sonia Alexandra Inc. and the co-founder, developer and president of TH Stone LLC, a globally recognized company with a worldwide distribution and education network. Its Stone Therapy products are available to the spa, wellness, health and related industries.

In Boca Raton, Florida, Sonia now spends much of her time writing, consulting, developing new products and facilitating workshops worldwide. As a continuing education provider, she travels nationally and internationally to teach and to share her vision.

www.Stone-Healing.com

* * *

Modern day "pseudoscience" crystal power is attempting to harness the energy in crystals recognizing the powerful connection between mind and matter.

* * *

The mood for holistic self-preservation, which so recently has become a favored route of self-fulfillment in the West, has always been the unquestioned way of life in the East.

* * *

EASY - TO - ORDER FORM

Audio and E-book formats are also available.

E-mail: Sonia@Stone-Healing.com
Fax: 1-561-361-3965 with this form
Phone: 1-866-680-5149 toll-free
Mail: Sonia Alexandra
         4521 North Dixie Highway
         Boca Raton, FL 33431

_____ Copies *The Art of Stone Healing* $15.99 Each
_____ Subtotal
_____ Sales tax 6.0% for shipments to Florida
_____ Shipping: within U.S. $4.50 for first book
             + $2.00 for each additional book
_____   outside U.S. $9.50 for first book
             + $5.00 for each additional book
_____ TOTAL Amount Due

We accept payment by credit card or money order
___Visa ___ MasterCard ___ American Express

Card   Exp.
Number_____ Date _____

Name on Card (please print) _____

Sonia Alexandra is an international facilitator and speaker in the spa and wellness industry. For workshops, seminars, individual sessions or speaking engagements, or for any personal communication, please contact her by any of the above order methods.